WA
235

D0495795

Professional Practice for Foundation Doctors

Titles in the Series

Health, Behaviour and Society: Clinical Medicine in Context	ISBN 9780857254610
Law and Ethics in Medical Practice	ISBN 9780857250988
Succeeding in your Medical Degree	ISBN 9780857253972

To order, please contact our distributor: BEBC Distribution, Albion Close, Parkstone, Poole, BH12 3LL. Telephone: 0845 230 9000, email: learningmatters@bebc.co.uk.
You can also find more information on each of these titles and our other learning resources at www.learningmatters.co.uk

Professional Practice for Foundation Doctors

Editors: Judy McKimm and Kirsty Forrest

Series Editors:
Judy McKimm, Kirsty Forrest and Aidan Byrne

NORTH HAMPSHIRE HOSPITAL HEALTHCARE
LIBRARY

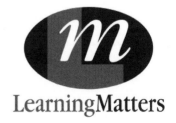
LearningMatters

First published in 2011 by Learning Matters Ltd

All rights reserved. No part of this publication may be reproduced, stored in a retrieval system or transmitted in any form by any means, electronic, mechanical, photocopying, recording, or otherwise, without prior permission in writing from Learning Matters.

© 2011 Introduction – Judy McKimm and Kirsty Forrest; Chapter 1 – Stuart Carney; Chapter 2 – Clare Morris; Chapter 3 – Sam Held; Chapter 4 – Caroline Elton; Chapter 5 – Sue Lister; Chapter 6 – Nicola Cooper and Alison Cracknell; Chapter 7 – John Spencer; Chapter 8 – John Spencer; Chapter 9 – Lai Fong Chiu and Laura Stroud; Chapter 10 – Stuart Anderson; Chapter 11 – Dominic Bell; Chapter 12 – Dominic Bell; Chapter 13 – Jill Thistlethwaite; Chapter 14 – Judy McKimm; Chapter 15 – Clare Morris; Chapter 16 – Brian D. Nicholson; Chapter 17 – Sue Morgan and Liam Young; Chapter 18 – Charlie Cooper; Chapter 19 – Judy McKimm and Kirsty Forrest.

The rights of Judy McKimm, Kirsty Forrest, Stuart Carney, Clare Morris, Sam Held, Caroline Elton, Sue Lister, Nicola Cooper, Alison Cracknell, John Spencer, Lai Fong Chiu, Laura Stroud, Stuart Anderson, Dominic Bell, Jill Thistlethwaite, Brian D. Nicholson, Sue Morgan, Liam Young and Charlie Cooper to be identified as Authors of this Work (as listed above) have been asserted by them in accordance with the Copyright, Designs and Patents Act 1988.

British Library Cataloguing in Publication Data
A CIP record for this book is available from the British Library.

ISBN 978 0 85725 284 5

This book is also available in the following ebook formats:
Adobe ebook ISBN: 978 0 85725 286 9
EPUB ebook ISBN: 978 0 85725 285 2
Kindle ISBN: 978 0 85725 287 6

Cover and text design by Code 5 Design Associates
Project management by Swales & Willis, Exeter, Devon
Typeset by Swales & Willis Ltd, Exeter, Devon
Printed and bound in Great Britain by Short Run Press Ltd, Exeter, Devon

Learning Matters Ltd
20 Cathedral Yard
Exeter EX1 1HB
Tel: 01392 215560
info@learningmatters.co.uk
www.learningmatters.co.uk

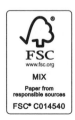

FSC
www.fsc.org
MIX
Paper from
responsible sources
FSC® C014540

Contents

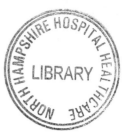

NORTH HAMPSHIRE HOSPITAL HEALTHCARE LIBRARY

Contents

Foreword from the Series Editors

The Learning Matters Medical Education Series

Medical education is currently experiencing yet another a period of change, typified in the UK with the introduction of the revised *Tomorrow's Doctors* (General Medical Council, 2009) and ongoing work on establishing core curricula for many subject areas. Changes are also occurring at Foundation and postgraduate levels in terms of the introduction of broader non-technical competencies, a wider range of assessments and revalidation requirements. This new series of textbooks has been developed as a direct response to these changes and the impact on all levels of medical education.

Research indicates that effective medical practitioners combine excellent, up-to-date clinical and scientific knowledge with practical skills and the ability to work with patients, families and other professionals with empathy and understanding, they know when to lead and when to follow and they work collaboratively and professionally to improve health outcomes for individuals and communities. In *Tomorrow's Doctors* (2009) the General Medical Council has defined a series of learning outcomes set out under three headings:

- Doctor as Practitioner

- Doctor as Scholar and Scientist

- Doctor as Professional

The books in this series do not cover practical clinical procedures or knowledge about diseases and conditions, but instead cover the range of non-technical professional skills (plus underpinning knowledge) that students and doctors need to know in order to become effective, safe and competent practitioners.

Aimed specifically at medical students (but also of use for junior doctors, teachers and clinicians), each book relates to specific outcomes of *Tomorrow's Doctors* (and where relevant the Foundation Curriculum), providing both knowledge and help to improve the skills necessary to be successful at the non-clinical aspects of training as a doctor. One of the aims of the series is to set medical practice within the wider social, policy and organisational agendas to help produce future doctors who are socially aware and willing and prepared to engage in broader issues relating to healthcare delivery.

Individual books in the series outline the key theoretical approaches and policy agendas relevant to that subject, and go further by demonstrating through case studies and scenarios how these theories can be used in work settings to achieve best practice. Plenty of activities and self-assessment tools throughout the book will help the reader to hone their critical thinking and reflection skills.

Chapters in each of the books follow a standard format. At the beginning a box highlights links to relevant competencies and outcomes from *Tomorrow's Doctors* and other medical curricula if appropriate. This sets the scene and enables the reader to see exactly what will be covered. This is extended by a chapter overview which sets out the key topics and what the student should expect to have learnt by the end of the chapter.

There is at least one case study in each chapter which considers how theory can be used in practice from different perspectives. Activities are included which include practical tasks with learning points, critical thinking research tasks and reflective practice/thinking points. Activities can be carried out by the reader or with others and are designed to raise awareness, consolidate understanding of theories and ideas and enable the student to improve their practice by using models, approaches and ideas. Each activity is followed by a brief discussion on issues raised. At the end of each chapter, a chapter summary provides an aide-memoire of what has been covered.

All chapters are evidence based in that they set out the theories or evidence that underpins practice. In most chapters, one or more 'What's the evidence' boxes provide further information about a particular piece of research or a policy agenda through books, articles, websites or policy papers. A list of additional readings is set out under the 'Going further' section, with all references collated at the end of the book.

The series is edited by Professor Judy McKimm, Dr Kirsty Forrest, and Dr Aidan Byrne, all of whom are experienced medical educators and writers. Book and chapter authors are drawn from a wide pool of practising clinicians and educators from the UK and internationally.

About the Authors

Stuart Anderson is Associate Dean of Studies at the London School of Hygiene and Tropical Medicine. He was previously senior lecturer in organisational behaviour in healthcare at the School, and is a former academic director of the NHS Service Delivery and Organisation (SDO) Research Programme. He originally qualified as a pharmacist, and his previous posts include principal pharmacist at Alder Hey Children's Hospital, Liverpool, chief pharmacist at Westminster Hospital, London and director of pharmacy at St George's Hospital, London. He is a Fellow of the Royal Pharmaceutical Society and of the Higher Education Academy. He is involved in the development of masters' and doctoral programmes in health leadership.

Dominic Bell is an intensive care consultant in Leeds. He holds a degree in Medical Law, sits as founder member of the Trust Ethics Committee and has written editorials, chapters and reviews on patient safety and ethical and legal matters within medicine. He has been specialty advisor to the NPSA and GMC and represented the Intensive Care Society on ethico-legal working parties. He acts as adviser to the Official Solicitor, assisting the Court in end-of-life decision-making, treatment decisions for patients with mental health disorders, and mediating between hospital staff and next-of-kin. He acts as independent expert at inquests and in police investigations into gross negligence manslaughter. He was appointed Assistant Deputy Coroner in 2009.

Stuart Carney is a psychiatrist and the Deputy National Director of the UK Foundation Programme Office. As a clinical advisor to the Medical Education and Training Programme Team at the Department of Health since 2004, he has helped shape the Foundation Programme with particular responsibility for coordinating the consistent delivery of the curriculum and academic training. He was Director of the Leicestershire, Northamptonshire and Rutland Foundation School between 2005 and 2009. Stuart is a Fellow of the Academy of Medical Educators.

Lai Fong Chiu has a background in public health, health promotion and health service management, and is currently a Senior Research Fellow at the Institute of Health Sciences, University of Leeds leading on teaching and research in health promotion. She is the originator and developer of the Community Health Educator Model (Health Promotion) for public health which has been adopted widely across the UK. She has published academic papers, book chapters and training and health education materials on cancer screening, minority ethnic communities and low-income groups. She is a member of the panel of referees for three NHS research programmes and a member of advisory panels on many research projects. She was on the editorial board of *Electronic Health* between 2005 and 2007, and associate editor (Health) of the *Action Research Journal* from 2007 to 2010. Lai Fong is regularly invited to speak at national and international conferences, at meetings of expert networks, is an advisory member of the WHO Task Force on Migrant Friendly and Culturally Competent Hospitals and co-ordinator of its working group on Patient and Community Empowerment.

Charlie Cooper has been an Associate Postgraduate Dean since 1999 and is a consultant in Intensive Care and Anaesthesia at Chesterfield Royal Hospital. He is a GMC Quality Panel Chair (Visits, Curriculum, and Certification), an elected council member of the Society for Education in Anaesthesia (UK), a faculty member of the Royal College of Anaesthetists (RCoA) 'Anaesthetist as

Educator' programme and the educationalist to the RCoA's Staff and Associate Specialist Committee. His special interests are the quality management of postgraduate medical education, the 'doctor in difficulty', assessment and feedback and professional development.

Nicola Cooper is a Consultant Physician/Honorary Senior Lecturer and Clinical Lead for Acute Medicine at St James's University Hospital in Leeds, UK, one of the largest teaching hospitals in Europe. A founder member of the hospital's patient safety programme, she is a Fellow of the NHS Institute's Improvement Faculty, and the Academy of Medical Educators. She is involved on a day-to-day basis in educating and supervising medical students and junior doctors and is the author/editor of a number of educational articles and textbooks.

Alison Cracknell is a Consultant in Medicine for Older People, at St James's University Hospital in Leeds. She has a clinical and academic interest in patient safety and service improvement. She has published on the incidence and preventability of adverse events in UK hospitals, and leads the novel spiral undergraduate patient safety curriculum at Leeds University Medical School. She is a member of the Health Innovation and Education Cluster for Patient Safety (Yorkshire and Humber), developing multi-professional postgraduate training and action for patient safety. She is also the British Geriatric Society Lead for patient safety.

Caroline Elton is a chartered psychologist with a special interest in career counselling and medical education. Originally trained as a secondary school science teacher, Caroline switched career direction and completed a PhD in the Department of Academic Psychiatry, Middlesex Hospital. Having changed career herself she became interested in career issues, and she undertook further training in both career and psychodynamic counselling. Caroline was an education adviser with KSS Deanery for ten years, and together with her colleague Joan Reid she wrote the career development handbook, 'ROADS to Success'. Whilst at KSS she was also involved with the initial development of the national medical careers website, and establishing the Postgraduate Certificate in Managing Medical Careers. In 2008 she joined London Deanery to head up the newly established Careers Unit.

Kirsty Forrest is a consultant anaesthetist at Leeds General Infirmary and Clinical Education Advisor at the Yorkshire and Humber Deanery. She is a regular teacher of both undergraduate students and postgraduate trainees. She is co-author and editor of a number of best-selling medical textbooks. Her academic interests are in skills training, student support and apprenticeship. She is co-academic lead for the Research, Evaluation and Special Studies strand of the Leeds medical undergraduate curriculum. Her other main interest is in developing teaching skills in others by directing and educating on courses for the Royal College of Anaesthetists (RCoA) and the Royal College of Surgeons and being an active member on the RCoA 'anaesthetists as educator' committee.

Sam Held is Patient and Family Services Manager at North Shore Hospice, Auckland. Sam's background in the public and voluntary sectors provides wide experience in working both within and across health, social care and community development boundaries, developing partnerships and introducing complex systemic change. Sam has taught in Further and Adult Education and, more recently, in higher and health professionals' education on leadership development; change management; user involvement; commissioning; strategic planning; managing staff and volunteers and project implementation. He is a qualified counsellor, is in advanced training as a transactional analysis psychotherapist and is actively involved in the Anglican Church.

Sue Lister is a Senior Lecturer in the Faculty of Health and Life Sciences at Coventry University, England and Senior Teaching Fellow with the NHS Institute for Innovation and Improvement. Sue's expertise is in quality management and service improvement from the patients' perspective. While on a full-time secondment to the NHS Institute, Sue implemented a project to introduce service improvement into the curriculum of pre-registration education of health and social care professionals. The programme was introduced into 50 universities in England which started a series of individual improvement projects being undertaken by at least 10,000 students per year. Her particular expertise is in making small changes that have a big impact.

Judy McKimm is Dean and Professor of Medical Education at Swansea University and Visiting Professor of Healthcare Education and Leadership at the University of Bedfordshire. She is a Senior Fellow of the Higher Education Academy and Fellow of the Academy of Medical Educators. Whilst at Imperial College School of Medicine, she co-ordinated the development and implementation of a new six-year MBBS/BSc programme. She has developed, implemented and evaluated many successful postgraduate faculty development programmes for medical and healthcare educators, leaders and advanced practitioners. Judy regularly speaks at national and international conferences, researches and publishes on medical and healthcare education and leadership. Since 1987, she has worked on international health reform, capacity building, quality assurance, professional licensing and education/training projects in many transition and former Soviet Union countries and, most recently, in Australia, New Zealand and Samoa.

Sue Morgan has a portfolio career. She works as an Associate Specialist in Elderly Care Medicine, Chairing the British Geriatric Staff and Associate Specialist (SAS) Group. She holds the educational portfolio for the SAS Working Group of the Royal College of Physicians and works as a Mentor and Facilitator for the London Deanery. The other part of her life is spent as a Senior Medical Assessor for the Medicines and Healthcare Products Regulatory Agency. She is a Medical Expert for the European Medicines Evaluation Agency and an Advisor and Reviewer for the BMJ. She is active in undergraduate, postgraduate and SAS Education.

Clare Morris is Associate Dean of the Postgraduate Medical School, University of Bedfordshire and course lead for the MA in Medical Education and linked awards in Dental Education, Medical Education Leadership and Medical Simulation. She has been involved in faculty development in medicine and health for the past 20 years and has a particular interest in how learning is supported in clinical workplaces.

Brian D. Nicholson is a GP Registrar based in York, with academic interests in epidemiology, health inequalities, and improving service delivery. He has conducted research into brain cancer epidemiology in teenagers and young adults, TB amongst migrant men in Kathmandu, and the use of Computed Tomography in bowel cancer diagnosis. Having founded the Alma Mata Global Health Network, he has a keen interest in international health, and works as a research assistant for the Nuffield Centre for International Health and Development. He plans to work in the developing world in a split clinical and academic role after completing training.

John Spencer is Professor of Primary Care and Clinical Education at Newcastle University, a Fellow of the Academy of Medical Educators, and a part-time GP. He has been involved in healthcare education for nearly 30 years, mostly undergraduate medical but also other disciplines, pre- and post-registration and CPD. He has been an active researcher and scholar in the field, was awarded the inaugural President's Silver Medal by the Academy of Medical Educators in 2009, and was Deputy Editor of Medical Education and Editor in Chief of *The Clinical Teacher* between 1998 and 2009.

Laura Stroud is Associate Director of Learning and Teaching for the School of Medicine, Leeds University. She is co-academic lead for the Research, Evaluation and Special Studies strand of the medical undergraduate curriculum and leads on undergraduate teaching in Public Health on behalf of the Academic Unit of Public Health. Laura has previously worked in the Voluntary Sector and has extensive experience of local health service strategic bodies as an independent member and Chair.

Jill Thistlethwaite is Professor of Medical Education and Director of the Centre for Medical Education Research and Scholarship at the University of Queensland in Brisbane, and a practising general practitioner. She has previously worked in clinical education and health professional education research at Warwick Medical School and the University of Sydney. She is a fellow of the Royal College of General Practitioners (UK), the Royal Australian College of General Practitioners and the Higher Education Academy. Her PhD from the University of Maastricht focused on shared decision-making and medical education and she has published widely on consultation skills, professionalism and interprofessional education. She is associate editor of the *Journal of Interprofessional Care* and the *Clinical Teacher*. Her research interests include collaborative practice, professionalism, patients as educators and revalidation.

Liam Young is a junior doctor in foundation year two who prior to medical school was a psychiatric nurse for many years, latterly working as the deputy manager of the South Islington Crisis Resolution Team. Liam worked in Crisis Resolution Teams for a number of years and has an extensive interest in the organisation and provision of mental health services. He plans to return to psychiatry and a well-organised life soon.

Acknowledgements

We would like to thank our fellow authors for their thoughtful contributions to the book, together with all those colleagues and students who have helped to shape our views of professional practice for junior doctors. On a more personal level we would also like to thank our respective partners Sam and Derek, for their constant love, support and encouragement.

Introduction: Generic Aspects of Professional Practice for Foundation Stage and Specialty Doctors
Judy McKimm and Kirsty Forrest

This book is designed to support trainee doctors during the Foundation and Specialty Stages of postgraduate training, including preparation and application for Specialty Training posts. It covers key areas in the generic (non-clinical) aspects of postgraduate education, training and professional development. This book makes explicit for new and continuing postgraduate trainees how the 'generic skills' fit into professional practice and development and how the knowledge base provided by the book underpins professional practice.

In summary, the book:

- assists the development of the knowledge, skills and competences required for good medical practice;

- addresses key areas within the 'generic', non-clinical elements and competences in the Foundation Programme and Speciality Curricula to support professional practice;

- uses case studies, activities and policy examples to illustrate key learning points;

- provides up-to-date information, reflects current policy developments and links to a range of useful information sources.

Generic competencies and skills

The Foundation Curriculum (FC) was introduced in 2007. Trainees have to achieve the specified competences in order to progress to the Specialty Training stage. This book enables trainees to develop their understanding of the FC competences – and the skills and behaviours required for good practice. It is also a useful resource for all those involved in Foundation training programmes such as clinical tutors and educational supervisors. There is evidence that many of those in support roles are still struggling to make sense of the new process, having trained under a very different system.

In 2008 and 2009, new competencies were produced for Academic Foundation Training posts which include teaching, research and leadership and management skills. These are also included throughout the book. In addition, all Specialty curricula are in the process of being revised to embed generic competencies and knowledge. Some Specialty trainees' undergraduate training did not focus specifically on generic skills and they also did not receive as much support as required in their Foundation training. This book helps to address these needs. Throughout the book, content is mapped against key areas identified in the non-clinical elements of the Foundation Programme Curriculum (UK Foundation Programme Office, 2010), the Academic 'Rough Guide' (UK Foundation Programme Office, 2008), the Compendium of Academic Competencies (UK Foundation Programme Office, 2009) and the generic competencies identified in specialty curricula.

In addition to changes in postgraduate curricula and associated training programmes, the General Medical Council has shifted emphasis in *Tomorrow's Doctors* (GMC, 2009), which sets the scene for basic medical training. The new approach is centred around three core attributes: Doctor as Practitioner; Doctor as Professional; and Doctor as Scholar and Scientist. *Tomorrow's Doctors* (2009) also emphasises the importance of patient safety and the quality of healthcare as a core thread that should run through professional practice.

In his introduction to the launch of *Tomorrow's Doctors* (2009), Professor Peter Rubin (Chair of the GMC Education Committee commented:

> For this edition, among a number of important changes, we have responded specifically to concerns about scientific education, clinical skills, partnership with patients and colleagues, and commitment to improving healthcare and providing leadership. We have also set out standards for the delivery of medical education with a new emphasis on equality and diversity, involving employers and patients, the professional development of teaching staff, and ensuring that students derive maximum benefit from their clinical placements.
>
> Today's undergraduates – tomorrow's doctors – will see huge changes in medical practice. There will be continuing developments in biomedical sciences and clinical practice, new health priorities, rising expectations among patients and the public, and changing societal attitudes. Basic knowledge and skills, while fundamentally important, will not be enough on their own. Medical students must be inspired to learn about medicine in all its aspects so as to serve patients and become the doctors of the future. With that perspective and commitment, allied to the specific knowledge, skills and behaviours set out in Tomorrow's Doctors and Good Medical Practice, they will be well placed to provide and to improve the health and care of patients.
>
> (General Medical Council, 2009)

The changes set out in *Tomorrow's Doctors* (2009) will play out in the postgraduate arena over the next few years. This book reflects this shift by placing emphasis on policy and strategy agendas, health systems, management and leadership of contemporary healthcare delivery. These areas are traditionally underrepresented in undergraduate medical curricula, yet increasingly emphasised in standards for assessing professional practice (e.g. in *Tomorrow's Doctors*, 2009) and in other guidance for medical schools and postgraduate providers such as the *Medical Leadership Competency Framework* (NHS Institute of Innovation and Improvement and Academy of Royal Colleges, 2010). The book also includes interpersonal aspects of 'professionalism' as well as a focus on how doctors need to collaborate effectively with others to improve patient care. Aspects such as patient safety, service improvement and health policy and management differentiate this book from others that focus either on clinical aspects or on more detailed generic skills.

Finally, the book provides guidance on research skills and contemporary learning and teaching approaches that may be useful to both trainees and their tutors/supervisors. These include, for example, reflective practice/critical reflection, portfolio development, mentoring and coaching. These topics are now being emphasised at undergraduate levels and reflected in the Foundation Curriculum, Academic Curriculum and Specialty curricula.

Book structure

The book is structured in six parts, each of which has a small number of chapters covering different topics:

- Your professional development
- Putting the patient first and improving services
- Management, legal and ethical frameworks
- Working collaboratively
- Teaching and research skills
- Working effectively as a professional.

Part 1 Your professional development

The first part is about contextualising trainees' education and training within a broader approach to professional and career development. It begins with an overview of the FT generic curriculum, academic curriculum and brief summary of Specialty generic curricula. It then looks at how trainees can best develop effective approaches to learning through an exploration of the different approaches on offer the support available. The section then considers different ways in which self-awareness and understanding can be enhanced introducing a range of tools and techniques. Finally, a systematic approach to planning career development is considered, including assessing training and development needs, how CVs can be enhanced, preparing and applying for Specialty training posts and resolving personal difficulties.

Part 2 Putting the patient first and improving services

The second part of the book takes a service improvement approach to professional practice, centred around the concept of putting the patient first and explaining the significant policy and strategy influences that drive service change and improvement.

The section considers clinical governance and quality improvement structures and processes and how postgraduate trainees can contribute towards these initiatives. Chapter 6 explores patient safety and the role of the healthcare team in reducing risk and error, considering roles of team member and leader and team dynamics. We then go on to look at the role of patients, carers and service users as contributors to healthcare and health improvement, considering diversity issues, cultural expectations, communications, expectations, rights and the role of the doctor as health advocate. Finally, we look at promoting health and the social context of healthcare, the influence of demographics on the patient population and health workforce, community engagement and empowerment, facilitating behaviour change through health education and promotion as part of public health priorities and national service frameworks.

Part 3 Management, legal and ethical frameworks

The third section of the book moves on to looking at health structures and systems at national, regional and organisational levels in the light of current policy and service agendas including the integrated service and personalisation agendas. We consider health management systems, including finance, management roles and functions, computing systems. We then go on to explore key elements of the legal framework and ethical principles that underpin professional medical practice. Taking the GMC's guidance in *Good Medical Practice* (GMC, 2006) we explore the legal responsibilities of trainees and how these dovetail with professional regulation and expectations, patients' rights and ethical principles, dilemmas and key cases.

Part 4 Working collaboratively

Doctors are members of health and social care teams who are required to work closely and effectively with managers, patients, patient groups and others. We explore the nature of effective collaboration by looking at interprofessional team-working and communication, emotional intelligence and developing self-awareness. We then look more closely at the nature of interprofessional working, professional roles and responsibilities and managing difficult situations. Finally, we consider how different leadership and management styles and approaches can help trainees to lead and manage change and innovation in relation to health services. We take a case study approach to exploring organisational, project and change management tools and techniques.

Part 5 Teaching and research skills

The range of career options for doctors includes academic roles in education, training and research. In addition to these specific career pathways, the majority of practising doctors have responsibility for juniors and sometimes medical students and there is increased recognition that teaching and research skills can and should be learned. We provide an overview of teaching and learning approaches, methods and techniques both at the 'bedside' and in the classroom, as well as looking at assessment, feedback and evaluation. We also take an overview of research skills and methodology, including audit, ethics applications, critical appraisal skills, project design and evaluation. This section will be particularly relevant to trainees on academic pathways.

Part 6 Working effectively as a professional

The final section brings together some of the themes of the book by looking at two related aspects of self-management: managing your time and workload and relating this to others' work priorities and managing yourself. In considering self-management, we look at how trainees need to take personal responsibility for their behaviour, recognise signs of positive and negative stress and know when and who to ask for help.

Learning features

Each chapter follows a similar format with a chapter overview, then the core text followed by a summary and further reading. References are summarised at the end of the book. Each chapter begins with contextualising the topic within the broad policy context (highlighting key national agendas for change or innovation) and the health system or organisational context, setting out why this issue is important and summarising key pieces of evidence.

Key issues for professional practice are then explored through case studies (from the perspective of the junior doctor, other health or social care professional, patient, carer or manager) and activities. Activities include practical tasks with feedback or learning points, critical thinking or research tasks and reflective practice/thinking points. Activities can be carried out by yourself or with others, these are designed to raise awareness, consolidate your understanding of theories and ideas and enable you to improve your practice using models, approaches and ideas. Each chapter highlights links to relevant Foundation competencies and outcomes, the full mapping of chapter context is available in an appendix to the book.

part 1

Your Professional Development

chapter 1

An Overview of the Foundation Programme
Stuart Carney

Chapter overview

The Foundation Programme transformed the first two years of postgraduate medical education in the UK. It has two broad objectives:

- to enable you to consolidate, develop and demonstrate the generic professional skills necessary for safe and effective patient care;
- to support you as you make informed decisions about your future medical career with advice, information and direct experience in a range of specialties and settings.

Central to this stage of training is the Foundation Programme Curriculum (the Curriculum), which sets out the learning outcomes expected of you. In addition to focusing on the care of the acutely ill patient, the Curriculum highlights the importance of generic skills such as professionalism, team-working and lifelong learning. However, the Foundation Programme is not just about ensuring that you are competent but should also enable you to excel. The Compendium of Academic Competencies provides a framework for you to move beyond 'good-enough' and develop your knowledge and skills as clinical leaders, educators and researchers.

This chapter sets out the rationale for reforming the first two years of postgraduate medical education. It focuses on the generic professional skills expected of all medical graduates, how you can develop these skills in the Foundation Programme and the importance of maintaining them throughout your career.

After reading this chapter you will be able to:

- discuss the rationale for including generic learning outcomes in the Curriculum;
- outline the key generic outcomes covered in the Curriculum;
- outline the opportunities for developing additional outcomes drawing on the Compendium of Academic Competences;
- describe how you can consolidate and develop the generic outcomes necessary for professional practice;
- describe how the assessment programme enables you to demonstrate that you have acquired and maintained generic outcomes;
- discuss the importance of these generic outcomes in your specialty training and continued professional development.

The foundations of professional practice

What is the Foundation Programme?

The Foundation Programme provides a bridge between medical school and specialty training (see Figure 1.1). Introduced in 2005, it transformed the first two years of postgraduate training. The Foundation Programme was part of a series of changes ushered in under the banner of 'Modernising Medical Careers' (MMC). These changes aimed to improve patient safety and patient care by improving the effectiveness of healthcare teams and developing medical practitioners, who are accountable and sensitive to the needs of patients and the National Health Service.

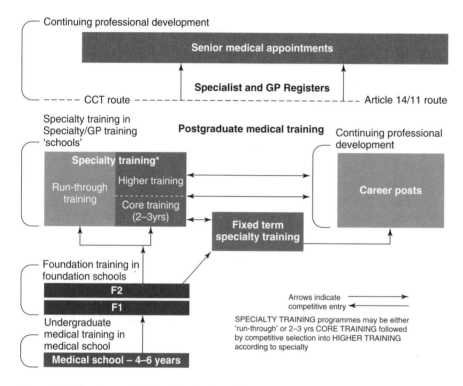

Figure 1.1 The shape of UK medical education

Foundation training is delivered through 25 UK foundation schools. During your training, you are allocated an educational supervisor and are responsible for maintaining your e-portfolio. There is a detailed Curriculum setting out what is expected of you as you make the transition from student to employee. Assessments take place in the workplace and judgements about satisfactory completion of F1 and F2 are made against agreed national criteria.

You must satisfactorily complete the two-year programme to be eligible to progress into specialty training. But the Foundation Programme is not just about meeting clinical and professional outcomes, you should also use the first 16 months, before recruitment to specialty training opens, to explore different career options. Foundation training aims to enable you to:

- develop and gain confidence in your clinical skills, particularly when you are treating acutely ill patients so that you can reliably diagnose and care for seriously ill patients;

- display professional attitudes and behaviour in your clinical practice;

- demonstrate your competence in these areas through a thorough and reliable system of assessment;

- have the opportunity to explore a range of career opportunities through working in different settings and in different areas of medicine;

- complete the requirements for eligibility to apply for full registration with the General Medical Council at the end of the first year of the Foundation Programme (UK Foundation Programme Office, 2010).

The Curriculum uses a spiral model. That means that you are expected to demonstrate the same outcomes by the end of F2 as at the end of F1 but at a higher level of competence. Although the Programme focuses on the assessment and management of the acutely ill patient, you are also expected to demonstrate a range of generic skills including the ability to work as a member of a multidisciplinary team, use evidence and data for patient care, prescribe safely and work effectively across different settings.

Before describing these generic professional skills in more detail, it is worth reflecting on the rationale for reforming the early years of postgraduate training and focusing on generic competences in particular.

Why was the Foundation Programme introduced?

The Foundation Programme and the broader MMC reforms sought to address a number of deficiencies in the old-style Senior House Officer (SHO) training. These included:

- *poor job structure*: around half of SHO posts were not part of a training rotation and the quality of training within training rotations was indifferent;

- *difficulty in planning training*: lack of a defined end-point to SHO training with varying time spent in the SHO grade;

- *weak selection and appointment procedures*: these were perceived to be inefficient, expensive, not mapped to a person specification and possibly non-compliant with employment legislation;

- *inadequate supervision, assessment and appraisal*: lack of structured training programmes made it difficult to introduce robust appraisal and identify doctors in difficulty;

- *shortage of careers advice*: there was a need for improved careers advice and the opportunity to experience a range of career options early in training;

- *no national workforce planning*: there was a lack of national planning for the number of SHO posts and significant variation in competition ratios and shortages of applicants for general practice posts and consultant posts in some specialties;
- *uncertainty about the relevance of Royal College examinations*: there was a wide variation in pass rates for these examinations.

But perhaps the biggest driver for change was a widespread concern about patient safety. A number of peer-reviewed papers had highlighted opportunities to improve patient safety through better medical training. These included concerns about deficiencies in the recognition of acutely ill patients and prescribing (McQuillan et al., 1998; Vincent et al., 2001; Dean et al., 2002). It was estimated that half of adverse event were preventable and 0.4 per cent of prescriptions included a potentially serious error.

As a result, patient safety is at the heart of the Curriculum (see Chapter 4). During the two-year programme, you are expected to consolidate and develop the skills you learned at medical school. This requires that you not only consistently deliver high-quality care but also actively contribute to improvements in clinical services; for example, through audit. Chapter 5 provides more detailed information on audit and clinical governance.

The Foundation Programme, however, is only the beginning of your postgraduate medical career. There will be many advances in the practice of medicine during your career and changes in the way in which the health service is structured. You will need to develop a flexible approach to your career so you can respond to an ever-changing health environment. It is essential that you use this time to get into the habit of identifying your learning needs, developing your skills and demonstrating your competence. Your professional development will depend on a commitment to lifelong learning, career development and reflection, all of which you can read more about in later chapters.

The Foundation Programme Curriculum

The Curriculum describes the outcomes expected of a foundation doctor completing the two-year programme. In addition, it outlines how you can develop your knowledge and skills and the range of workplace-based assessment tools in use.

Although the Curriculum focuses on the assessment and management of the acutely ill patient, it also draws attention to the importance of managing patients with chronic health conditions. Chronic health conditions often co-exist with acute illness and account for the majority of all clinical consultations.

Patient safety and professional development are at the core of the Curriculum (Box 1.1). These underpin the generic professional competences that you are expected to acquire and demonstrate during the Programme. Generic professional competences include putting the patient first, improving services, teaching and working effectively as a professional. In addition, the Foundation Programme provides an opportunity for you to develop additional skills such as leadership/management and research skills. These core professional attributes are explored in greater detail in later chapters.

Key messages of the Foundation Programme Curriculum (AoMRC 2010)

Patient safety

- Patient safety must be put at the centre of healthcare.
- High-quality patient care depends, among other aspects of practice, on effective multi-disciplinary teams.

Personal development

- Learning in, and from, practice is the most effective way for professionals to develop most of their expertise.
- Doctors are committed to lifelong learning in, and from, the practice of medicine in the clinical environment and through repeated clinical experience. Foundation doctors will be expected to develop critical thinking and professional judgement, especially where there is clinical uncertainty.
- Every clinical experience is a learning opportunity and should be reflected upon from the perspective of developing skills, understanding, clinical acumen and performance.
- Failure to recognise this calls into question an individual's commitment to life-long learning and continuing professional development.
- Doctors must continuously work to improve performance, that is, improve what you actually do as distinct from your capabilities.

The compendium of academic competences

The Foundation Programme is not just about ensuring that you are competent but also about enabling you to excel. The UK Foundation Programme Office has developed a Compendium of Academic Competences (UK Foundation Programme Office, 2009). It provides a framework for you to develop your knowledge and skills as a clinical leader, educator and researcher.

The Compendium is not comprehensive or prescriptive but instead is designed to help you, in partnership with your supervisor, to select areas for your personal development. Although, it is expressed in terms of outcomes, it may not be possible for you to meet all (or any) of these outcomes but instead you could realistically develop the knowledge, understanding and some of the skills/competences underpinning the outcome. For example, while it may not be possible to write and submit an application for ethics approval, you may be able to learn about the legal framework underpinning ethics approval.

The Compendium is split into three sections: leadership and management, teaching outcomes and research outcomes. As you might expect, there is significant overlap between the sections; to be a good leader you will need to be able to critically appraise data and teach.

The leadership and management section is based on the *Medical Leadership Competency Framework* (the MLCF – produced jointly by the NHS Institute of Innovation and Improvement and Academy of Medical Royal Colleges in 2008 and revised in 2010). It builds on the generic leadership competences required of all foundation doctors set out in the Curriculum and focuses on five core areas.

- your personal qualities;
- working with others;
- managing services;
- improving services;
- setting direction.

Chapter 14 discusses clinical leadership and management ideas and case examples, focused on the MLCF. Similarly the teaching and research sections builds on the Curriculum. If you are interested in developing your teaching skills, the Academy of Medical Educators' Professional Standards document may also be of interest (Academy of Medical Educators, 2009). Chapter 15 provides more information on teaching skills and Chapter 16 gives you an introduction to research skills. Table 1.1 sets out the key outcomes described in the Compendium in the research section.

Table 1.1 Research outcomes

	Research planning	*Conduct of research*	*Dissemination*
Research skills	• Question formulation and literature searching • Critically appraise a topic • Systematically review a topic • Write a research proposal volunteers or NHS patients • Write an application for funding	• Carry out a lab-based experiment, analyse the results and write a report • Carry out a research study involving human • Carry out a population-based study, analyse the results and write a report	
Research governance	• Write an application for ethics approval	• Take informed consent for a research project	
Teaching and communication			• Write up a study for publication in a peer-reviewed journal • Present the results as a poster presentation • Present the results as an oral presentation

Consolidating and developing your generic competences

During both F1 and F2, you are required to provide evidence that you have met all of the outcomes set out in the Curriculum.

For each outcome, you should consider how you intend to acquire the knowledge and competences underpinning the outcome, how you will demonstrate that you have achieved and maintained the outcome and when you hope to demonstrate that you have met the outcome. Your e-portfolio has a personal development plan section which is based on the outcomes set out in the Curriculum. There will also be space for you to plan additional learning objectives.

Every clinical experience has the potential to be a learning opportunity. Your foundation school will allocate you to an educational and clinical supervisor and provide a generic training course but it is up to you to exploit every opportunity to develop your skills, understanding and performance. There is also a range of e-learning available and many hospitals provide access to clinical skills labs and other simulated environments. Chapter 2 shows you more about how to make the most of your learning in the Foundation Programme.

Demonstrating your generic competences

It is your responsibility to gather evidence that you have met, maintained and, if possible, exceeded the standard of competence expected of you during the Foundation Programme.

There are six workplace-based assessments tools used in the Foundation Programme:

- *Team Assessment of Behaviour (TAB)* – this is a multi-source feedback tool.

- *Logbook of Procedural Skills* – this tool should be used to provide evidence that you can competently perform all 15 procedures listed in the logbook by the end of F1.

- *Direct Observation of Procedural Skills (DOPS)* – you should use this tool to provide evidence that you can perform procedures not listed in the logbook.

- *Mini Clinical Evaluation Exercise (mini-CEX)* – like DOPS this tool is used to assess how you interact with patients.

- *Case-based Discussion (CbD)* – this tool provides an opportunity for you to discuss clinical cases with a senior colleague.

- *Educational Assessment Tool* – this tool should be used to assess your teaching skills.

Workplace-based assessments should not only provide an opportunity for you to gather evidence but should also provide you with constructive feedback. These assessment tools are all accessed through your e-portfolio.

You will be busy during your clinical placements and it is very tempting to delay undertaking the assessments until the end of the year. You should however space your assessments throughout the year to avoid struggling towards the end of the year. If you are having difficulties, it is important that you identify these early on in your training so that you can work with your clinical and educational supervisor(s) to improve your practice.

You should also collect other evidence in your e-portfolio. This can include audits, reflective learning reports, attendance at courses and letters or cards from patients.

The Foundation Programme is only the beginning

Throughout your professional career, you will need to develop and maintain these generic professional skills. Depending on your role and at different stages in your career, it is likely that some skills – for example, teaching or management – will be more prominent. However, irrespective of your role and chosen specialty there are a number of competences integral to being a doctor in the UK.

The Academy of Medical Royal Colleges has developed a Common Competences Framework for Doctors (CCFD) (Academy of Medical Royal Colleges, 2009). It is based on the four domains of the GMC's Framework for *Appraisal and Assessment*.

- Domain 1 Knowledge, Skills and Performance.

- Domain 2 Safety and Quality.

- Domain 3 Communication, Partnership and Teamwork.

- Domain 4 Maintaining Trust.

The CCFD is designed to be a reference document setting out the basic and generic competences required of a doctor without being specialty specific. It forms the basis of specialty training curricula and supports the spiral nature of learning that will underpin your continual development, from medical school, the Foundation Programme, specialty training and into your work as a specialist.

Chapter summary

This chapter has covered:

- why generic professional learning outcomes feature so prominently in the Foundation Programme Curriculum and your continued professional development;

- the key generic areas covered in the Foundation Programme Curriculum and the Compendium of Academic Competences;

- how you can consolidate, develop and demonstrate the generic outcomes during the Foundation Programme and beyond.

GOING FURTHER

More information about the Foundation Programme, including key documents, is available from the UKFPO website: **www.foundationprogramme.nhs.uk**

The *Medical Leadership Competency Framework* is available through the NHS Institute of Innovation and Improvement's website: **www.institute.nhs.uk**

The Professional Standards for Medical Educators is available through the Academy of Medical Educators' website: **www.medicaleducators.org**

Common Competences Framework for Doctors is available through the Academy of Medical Royal Colleges' website: **www.armrc.org.uk**

chapter 2

Developing Effective Approaches to Learning During Foundation Training
Clare Morris

Achieving foundation competences

This chapter will introduce you to the following syllabus and competences set out in the *Foundation Programme Curriculum* 2010.

Outcome 12 Maintaining good medical practice

12.1 Lifelong learning
Outcome: demonstrates the knowledge, attitudes, behaviours, skills and competences needed to start self-directed lifelong learning.

Competences: F1 and F2

- Learns from experience/experiential learning.
- Reviews professional learning needs and takes step to address these.
- Maintains a professional development portfolio by recording learning needs and reflections.
- Uses WPBAs (workplace-based assessments) and MSF (multisource feedback) to get feedback and improve performance.
- Recognises errors and mistakes and demonstrates measures to learn from them.
- Arranges and prepares for own appraisal in a timely manner.
- Contributes to the appraisal, assessment or review of students and other colleagues.

Assessment: CBD (case based discussion) and MSF.

Knowledge

- The concept of continuing professional development.
- The role of appraisal and revalidation.
- The purpose of assessment (formative and summative).

Chapter overview

The point at which you graduate from medical school signals an important transition: from student to doctor and lifelong learner. Formal curriculum structures, with timetabled teaching and high-stake summative assessments make way for the curriculum of the workplace. Here, learning arises through engagement in day-to-day work activity with formative assessment processes guiding and evidencing your progress. Learning to learn in these new conditions is an important part of this transition. This chapter aims to guide you through the first years of postgraduate training and equip you to make the most of learning opportunities arising throughout your medical career.

After reading this chapter you will be able to:

- recognise the learning opportunities arising in day-to-day work;
- appreciate the educational value and effective use of workplace-based assessments (WPBA);
- discriminate between descriptive and reflective accounts of practice and feel better equipped for the latter;
- differentiate between key terms used to describe learning and assessment in postgraduate medical education.

Context: a modernised medical curriculum

In 2005, postgraduate medical education underwent a period of significant reform under the auspices of Modernising Medical Careers (MMC). New curriculum models were introduced which offered more closely structured training periods, more formalised supervisory processes and a range of WPBA tools to guide and evidence progress. Attention has turned to the continuing professional development of all doctors, linked to new processes of licensing and revalidation. All doctors are expected to learn through working and evidence this learning; the extent to which you are prepared for this challenge is open to question. A GMC-commissioned study on preparedness for practice notes that

> new doctors were not able to predict some areas in which they were underprepared, as these only became apparent after working. These included adapting to hospital procedures, clarifying the role of an F1 and understanding the boundaries of that role.
>
> (Illing et al., 2008, pii)

The study also flags up new graduates' concerns about dealing with acutely ill patients, managing their workloads and performing practical procedures in real life, rather than in simulation. This chapter aims to prepare you to make the most of the learning opportunities arising from and structured around workplace-based learning in undergraduate and foundation years. This means shifting attention from teaching (and teachers) to your own learning. To start this process let us begin with a case study of medical student learning in the workplace.

Learning in the workplace

Case study 2.1: Two medical students' accounts of the same clinical attachment

Andy

Really busy setting – loads going on all the time so lots of opportunities for hands-on experience. Let me do lots of things when I asked, so I developed skills in venepuncture, catheterisation, suturing and reading X-rays (which I could also brush up in the skills lab). The nurses and F2s were really helpful here – and gave me some honest feedback when asked. I chose to attend some ward rounds and meetings which gave me a better idea of how the hospital works and made me feel more part of the team. I joined the protected teaching time for the F1s as well and one of them let me shadow them on nights, which was a real eye opener. The consultant-led teaching was excellent, but I would have welcomed more opportunities to ask questions and get some feedback on my progress.

Steve

It is a really busy place with lots of trainees – to be honest I didn't feel as if there was much time left for medical student teaching. We did have some excellent teaching sessions from the Consultant and I joined the protected teaching time for the F1s. I also spent a lot of time in the skills lab, brushing up my techniques for the OSCEs. The hospital library is fantastic too – so rather than hang around with nothing to do I got some really good revision done for finals. I did get a bit of hands-on experience, but not as much as I would have liked.

Whilst Andy and Steve were together on the same clinical placement, their accounts differ. Andy places value in being part of a team, learning through hands-on experience and being guided by different members of the team. This type of learning has been described as *learning-as-participation*, where the goal of learning is to become a full participant in the activities of the workplace (Sfard, 1998). Steve, on the other hand, places value in formal teaching and learning opportunities, linked to forthcoming examinations. This type of learning has been described as *learning-as-acquisition*, where the goal of learning is the accumulation of knowledge and skills (Sfard, 1998). Both have their place in medical education and training; however, problems arise when only one type is recognised or valued by learners or teachers. Arguably, Andy's orientation to learning will stand him in good stead for foundation years; he is focused on making the most of everyday learning opportunities, actively seeks these out and recognises that his 'teachers' are many. Andy also recognises that valuable learning goes beyond the acquisition of skills to encompass a broader understanding of organisational and working practices. Steve seems to miss these implicit learning opportunities, but he is not alone in this. Recent studies of the perceived educational value of 'rounds' reveal the different perceptions of trainers and trainees. The former (Andy) placed value in role modelling, peer learning and significant event analysis, the latter (Steve) desired more formal teacher-led sessions (Swanwick and Morris, 2010).

Being able to make the 'implicit explicit' is an invaluable skill for new doctors. Eraut (2000) makes helpful distinctions between different types of what he calls 'non-formal' learning, based on learning intent. At one level there is *implicit learning*: the type of learning that goes unnoticed but unconsciously influences our future actions. At the other end of the scale is *deliberative learning*, where time is deliberately set aside for learning. In between these two extremes we have *reactive learning* where learning that arises spontaneously is recognised and made explicit to oneself at the time. Steve and Andy both demonstrate intent to learn deliberatively, Andy is perhaps more prepared for emergent learning opportunities associated with reactive learning. Both are essential orientations to learning in the foundation years.

ACTIVITY 2.1 EXPLORING INFORMAL LEARNING

Go to the Infed website **www.infed.org/biblio/inf-lrn.htm** and read the article about informal learning, paying particular attention to ideas around non-formal and situated learning

Identify at least three ways in which these ideas are potentially relevant to guide your engagement with workplace-based learning in the foundation years.

Learning in the foundation years

Chapter 1 gives an overview of the Foundation Programme and the Foundation Programme website provides you with all the detail you will need about the teaching, learning and assessment during the first two years. You can download copies of the Foundation Programme Curriculum, Reference Guide and Rough Guides from **www.foundationprogramme.nhs.uk**

Figure 2.1 provides a visual overview of a typically structured year.

In the following sections we will explore the thinking behind the foundation curriculum tools and processes. This will include: the use of an e-portfolio; the value of WPBA; making the most of supervision sessions and developing reflective practice. In order to make sense of the curriculum however, you will need a grasp of some key educational concepts and ideas. Complete Activity 2.2 before moving forward with this chapter.

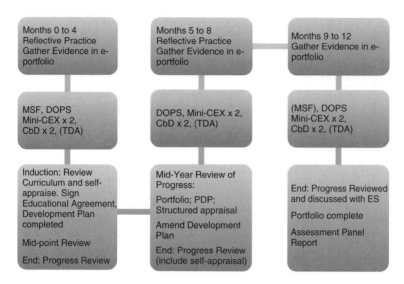

Figure 2.1 An overview of a typical foundation year

ACTIVITY 2.2 LEARNING THE LANGUAGE

Every professional discipline has its own language and terminology, and education is no exception. Table 2.1 contains some key terms and some simple definitions. Your task is to match the terms with their definitions. The key to answers at is the end of the chapter.

Table 2.1 Key terms and definitions

Terms		Definitions	
1	Appraisal	A	WPBA tool: clinical reasoning
2	CbD	B	WPBA tool: holisitic view of performance in workplace
3	Clinical Supervisor	C	Assessment FOR learning
4	Criterion Referenced	D	A measure of fitness for purpose of a particular assessment tool
5	Developing the Clinical Teacher	E	A developmental conversation designed to enhance subsequent performance
6	DOPS	F	A tool to record competence in carrying out specified procedures
7	Educational Supervisor	G	WPBA tool: observed clinical encounter
8	Feedback	H	A document to guide and record performance and progress over time
9	Formative assessment	I	Person(s) responsible for taking an overview of progress and providing structured review opportunities

10	Log book	J	WPBA tool: observed practical procedure and doctor–patient interaction
11	Mini-CEX	K	Assessment made against benchmarked pre-determined standards
12	MSF /TAB	L	Assessment OF learning
13	Norm Referenced	M	A process of identifying learning needs, negotiating learning outcomes and agreeing goals.
14	PDP	N	WPBA tool: teaching and/or presentation skills
15	Portfolio	O	A formalised review of progress with a designate ES and linked action planning
16	Reliability	P	Person(s) responsible for day-to-day supervision of practice
17	Summative assessment	Q	A measure of likely reproducibility of assessment outcomes
18	Validity	R	Assessment ranked against performance of others at similar stage of training

Personal development planning and the e-portfolio

One of the characteristic features of *reactive learning* is the learner's preparedness for emergent learning opportunities and the recognition of learning opportunities when they arise. In the case study, Andy saw possibilities in learning through shadowing a night shift, asked for feedback from the nurses who helped him learn new procedures and saw value in combining his hands-on experience with some skills lab practice. In a low-key way, Andy was able to recognise some of his learning needs, seek out opportunities for on-the-job learning and more deliberative learning. He also recognised the value of feedback and signalled desire for more input to help him judge his own progression. Andy demonstrates the value of a 'plan-do-review' cycle (see Figure 2.2) developed from Kolb's work on experiential learning (Kolb, 1984). It is easy to map the foundation year onto this cycle, and to identify the rich range of tools you will have to support your learning. You are not alone in this process – you will have an educational supervisor and clinical supervisors to support you – but the onus is upon you to make sure you structure and review your progress carefully.

Personal Development Planning, based on regular learning needs analysis, is key to this process. The goal is to identify specific learning needs that can be translated into your own learning outcomes. Identifying needs is an ongoing iterative process, informed by self-appraisal, formative assessment (assessment for learning), summative

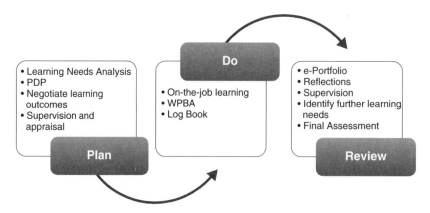

Figure 2.2 A plan-do-review cycle for foundation years

assessment (assessment of learning), appraisal and feedback from a range of sources. By having clear goals, you can avoid a 'scatter-gun' approach to your own development, actively seeking out the types of working and learning experiences that foster your development.

ACTIVITY 2.3 LEARNING NEEDS ANALYSIS

Drawing upon your most recent clinical experience, imagine you are an F2 and are asked to cover a shift for the CT1.

Other than flagging up professional issues of your readiness and appropriateness to cover and do a job you are not necessarily trained to do, what would be your most pressing learning needs in this scenario?

How do you know?
If you are unclear about your needs, what resources might you draw upon to become more informed?

Go back to Figure 2.1 and highlight the various ways in which learning needs identification and analysis happen implicitly and explicitly over a year.

The e-portfolio is designed to capture all aspects of the plan-do-review cycle. As such it is an important tool, which enables you to structure learning in the most opportunistic of environments. It works well as a formative assessment tool, drawing upon and triangulating evidence from a range of sources. WPBA is absolutely fundamental to this process; it offers formative assessment tools that can map your progression over the year and help you identify new learning needs at the same time. The next section explores their use in more detail.

What's the evidence? Use of e-portfolios

The foundation year's e-portfolio is designed to help you plan your learning, guide your development, evidence competence and record your progress. A recent systematic review of the effectiveness of portfolios for postgraduate assessment and development (Tochel et al., 2009) supports their use. They draw a number of conclusions that map well to the intended use of e-portfolios, linked assessment and supervisory practices. Specifically: the particular benefit of electronic (rather than paper-based) portfolios to encourage feedback and reflection; high-level organisational support to ensure uptake and sustainability; support of a well-informed mentor; triangulation of assessment methods with multiple raters and the increasing responsibility for learning fostered.

Workplace-based assessment

WPBA is perhaps the most misunderstood and maligned aspect of the Foundation Curriculum. Used well, WPBA tools have the potential to be powerful educational tools that can be used at all stages of the plan-do-review cycle. This means understanding the thinking behind them so you don't fall into a common trap of viewing them as summative, high-stakes assessment tools. WPBA tools are *formative*, providing structured opportunities to observe and review aspects of your performance across a range of different types of work activities. They are *learner-led*, which means you are responsible for selecting appropriate situations to be observed and suitable observers. If you select naturally occurring opportunities to be observed, you will ensure the *validity* of the tools. By ensuring a wide range of assessors you improve *reliability*. You are also responsible for using them wisely, spreading them out over the year. They provide *qualitative data* about your observed strengths and provide a *platform to discuss emerging development needs* and how to address them. All WPBA tools build in a requirement for *debrief and feedback*. They are also *norm referenced*, with the 'norm' being a typical foundation year doctor at the end of the relevant stage of training. So, in week one of your foundation year 1, your performance would be compared to that of a foundation year doctor who has completed the first year of training. By using this benchmark, you are able to *map and trace progression* over time. That is why the assessments should be spaced out over the year, rather than clustered towards the end of the year (as a traditional summative assessment might be). You do not have to 'pass' each individual assessment, but they are looked at cumulatively, alongside other evidences in your portfolio to *inform sign-off decisions*. See also the General Medical Council's guidance on Workplace Based Assessment, 2010c.

There are a large number of resources on the Foundation Programme website, which provide specific detail on each of the assessments, including frequency of use and timings over the year (see Figure 2.1 for a quick guide). There are six tools. Two tools are used to look at doctor–patient consultations: the *mini-CEX* (mini clinical examination) looks at clinical encounters, such as history taking, examination and consultations; the *DOPS* (Direct Observation of Procedural Skills) looks at performance of practical procedures, but with an emphasis on doctor–patient interaction. The *Logbook* is used to record achieved competences with specified procedural skills. A new assessment, *Developing the Clinical Teacher*, looks at your emerging abilities in teaching or giving a presentation. *CbD* (Case-based Discussion) is based on the American concept of chart-stimulated recall, and provides an opportunity to explore clinical reasoning. Cases are used as triggers for discussion, to extend your thinking about the work that you do. Finally, *TAB* (Team Assessment of Behaviour) is the preferred MSF (multi-source feedback) tool, providing a rich picture of your performance in the workplace, informed by all members of the team (including administrative staff, nursing staff, healthcare professionals and other medical staff). TAB is particularly helpful in identifying new doctors who may be in some difficulty and so for this reason it is best done in the first four months of the year so additional support may be put in place and progress reviewed in a timely manner.

Feedback is an important and integral aspect of each workplace-based assessment tool. Feedback at its best takes the form of a developmental conversation, where both parties critique performance (strengths as well as weaknesses), identify emergent needs, consider how best to achieve these and set goals for improvement. All supervisors should now be trained in how to facilitate an effective feedback session, but you can influence this process too. When you ask your assessor to observe you, give them some background information and steer them towards those aspects you would most like help with. For example, 'I have chosen this as an assessment opportunity as I really struggle to talk about the procedure and reassure the patient while actually doing the procedure. Feedback on my communication skills as well as technical skills would be really helpful' or 'I chose this case as it left me feeling unsettled and out of my depth. I would really value an opportunity to think it through, identify misunderstandings and work out how I could avoid a situation like that happening again.' By priming your observer, you are already displaying professional behaviour and attitudes and signalling expectations that you will engage in a shared dialogue.

What's the evidence? Assessment, feedback and performance

The Foundation Curriculum brings to the fore the importance of formative assessment; in other words, assessment-for-learning practices, aimed to enhance subsequent performance. A systematic review of the literatures on the relationship between assessment, feedback and physicians' clinical performance (Veloski et al., 2006) underlines this important relationship. Of the 41 studies meeting inclusion criteria, three-quarters demonstrated a positive effect for feedback alone.

Developing reflective practice

The e-portfolio and WPBA tools are designed to support the development of *reflective practice*. The term 'reflective practice' emerges from the work of John Dewey and

Donald Schön, and is used to capture types of professional thinking in and on action. Schön describes reflection-in-action as follows:

> The practitioner allows himself to experience surprise, puzzlement, or confusion in a situation which he finds uncertain or unique. He reflects on the phenomenon before him, and on the prior understandings which have been implicit in his behaviour. He carries out an experiment which serves to generate both a new understanding of the phenomenon and a change in the situation.
>
> (Schön, 1983, p68)

Reflection-on-action is a later, more deliberative process, where the practitioner rethinks the situation, exploring his or her feelings and responses and considering if change in practice is merited. This may be a solo pursuit (for example, as a reflective entry in an e-portfolio) or a shared endeavour, as part of a WPBA debrief, clinical or educational supervision session, or appraisal. Reflection is often presented as if it is a linear, structured process. In reality it is often cyclical and iterative. Figure 2.3 brings together a number of aspects of reflection (Jones, undated). Reflection often starts with a personal experience, an event, situation or issue that demands further thought (the 'I' aspect). Attending to this experience means being mindful of not only what happened, but also when and why. In thinking through the situation, you might also take time to consider what others might do, think or feel in the same situation (the 'we' aspect). To what extent is your response similar or different and what might you learn from them and vice versa? How would you have felt in the patient or carer's shoes? You may also wish to hold your response up to the wider community by engaging with literatures, policy guidelines, NICE (National Institute for Health and Clinical Evidence) guidelines and protocols (the 'they' aspect). Are there things you might have done differently? Can your experiences inform the development of organisational protocols for example? Reflection can be seen as a conversation with yourself, a process where you ask yourself questions and think through possible answers. The questioning approach enables you to move beyond descriptive accounts of what happened, into more reflective thought. By taking this questioning approach into supervision and appraisal situations, you can test out your thinking with others.

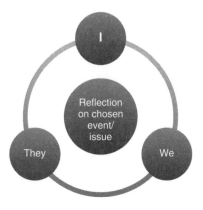

Figure 2.3 A reflective cycle

ACTIVITY 2.4 DEVELOPING REFLECTION

In the case study above, Andy and Steve both provide a clear *descriptive* account of their placement experiences. Andy describes his experience of shadowing a night shift as 'a real eye opener'. How might you help him develop this into a more reflective account, which explores the ways in which his 'eyes were opened'? Steve felt there 'was little time left for medical student teaching'. How might you help him reflect on opportunities for learning? For both, consider the types of questions you might want to ask them and the kinds of questions they might ask themselves, to develop a more reflective stance.

As a follow-up activity, visit the Patients Voices website (Patient Voice Programme, **www.patientvoices.org.uk**) and, in particular, the stories from Junior Doctors in Training. Listen to Matthew Critchfield's story called 'Yeah, I'll go' (**www. patientvoices.org.uk/flv/0257pv384.htm**). It is a good example of reflective thinking and may well prompt you to consider the ways in which the most powerful learning experiences are often the unplanned ones.

Making the most of supervision

The plan-do-review cycle can be used as a model to guide you through your foundation years. It can also guide your approach to supervision and appraisal sessions. Planning in this respect means keeping all documentation up to date in your e-portfolio. It also means doing some reviewing, looking over recent assessments and reflective entries to identify key areas of strength to date, as well as areas where you require more experience or have particular difficulties to address. It means thinking about what you would like to achieve from the supervision or appraisal situation and articulating these, before or at the start of the session. You should also make sure you are an 'expert' in your own curriculum. Many supervisors will support medical students, foundation doctors and doctors in specialty training. It is not reasonable to expect them to be fully conversant with every curriculum, you can act as a guide here.

The 'do' aspect is about taking an active role during the session, being reflective and receptive. It also means seeking particular guidance or feedback if not immediately offered by your supervisor. Reviewing is an important aspect of this process, engaging in a critical dialogue in order to recognise future development needs. Through review and discussion you can begin to plan for the next period of training, identifying short- and medium-term goals for your development. These can be linked to particular learning opportunities. Some will be deliberative learning experiences, drawing on available teaching sessions and learning resources. Some may require you to go beyond the workplace and engage with particular training courses or personal study activity. Many can be factored into day-to-day working experiences with some forethought. Don't restrict yourself to seeing your clinical supervisor as the only guide. Your peers, other doctors in training, nurses, healthcare professionals and patients themselves can guide your learning.

Build a review into your action plan. If you identify a need to develop your clinical reasoning, start thinking about an opportune moment to do a CBD. If you wish to develop consultation skills, think about using a mini-CEX or DOPS. Identify particular procedural skills to enhance and actively scan for opportunities to assist others doing them. Set yourself a goal to ensure you regularly reflect on experiences. In these ways, learning and supervision become an integral part of your ongoing professional development rather than add-ons to working life.

Chapter summary

- The transition from student to foundation doctor means a shift in thinking from teaching to learning, recognising that working and learning are integrally related.

- Being professional means taking responsibility for your own learning whilst working effectively with designated supervisors to identify learning needs, plan for your development and to monitor and review progress.

- The Foundation Curriculum offers a range of formative assessment tools and resources that support this process.

- Reflective practice is supported through active and purposeful engagement in supervision and appraisal processes.

GOING FURTHER

The London Deanery Faculty Development Unit offer free e-learning modules at **www.faculty.londondeanery.ac.uk/e-learning**. You will find useful resources on assessing educational needs, setting learning objectives, supervision, workplace-based assessment and appraisal. You may like to use these to follow up some of the issues raised in this chapter.

Key to Table 2.1 answers

1	2	3	4	5	6	7	8	9	10	11	12	13	14	15	16	17	18
O	A	P	K	N	J	I	E	C	F	G	B	R	M	H	Q	L	D

chapter 3

Understanding Yourself
Sam Held

Achieving foundation competences

This chapter will help prepare you for the Foundation Programme as a whole, but is particularly relevant to the following outcomes and competencies in the curriculum.

1.1 Behaviour in the workplace

- Always recognises own level of competence and asks for help from appropriate sources.
- Demonstrates the ability and habit of reflection on experience, as well as learning from practice, then instituting appropriate changes in this practice.
- Acts with empathy, honesty and sensitivity in a non-confrontational manner.
- Respects and supports the privacy and dignity of patients.
- Is courteous, polite and professional when communicating with both patients and colleagues.
- Has a non-judgemental approach.
- Is aware of patient expectations around personal presentation of doctors such as dress and social behaviour.
- In all interactions with both patients and colleagues takes account of factors pertaining to the patient's age, colour, culture, disability, ethnic or national origin, gender, lifestyle, marital or parental status, race, religion or beliefs, sexual orientation, or social or economic status (*The New Doctor*, GMC).

2.1 Eliciting a history

- Takes accomplished, concise, targeted history and communicates in complex situations, which include:

  - psychological (e.g. the patient is confused, has psychiatric/psychological problems which impact on physical health);
  - social and personal (e.g. English is not the patient's first language, impaired hearing/vision, learning difficulties);
  - the patient's personal factors (see The New Doctors' list in Professionalism).

- Takes account of background issues where relevant and appropriate, including verbal and non-verbal cues.

2.2 Examination

- Explains and gains appropriate consent for the examination procedure.
- Performs a mental state assessment.
- Demonstrates awareness of safeguarding children (Levels 1 and 2) and vulnerable adults.
- Asks for a chaperone where appropriate.
- Explains and gains appropriate consent for the examination procedure.
- Performs a mental state assessment.
- Demonstrates awareness of safeguarding children (Levels 1 and 2) and vulnerable adults.
- Asks for a chaperone where appropriate.

Chapter overview

How well do you know yourself? Quite probably a lot more than you did when you started studying medicine. It's a question many of us struggle with, as we try to work out how close we are to who we think we are, and who we would actually like to be. Another important question at certain key stages of our careers, and indeed our lives, is just how much does it matter?

The Foundation Curriculum competencies listed above includes those where a good insight into what makes you tick as an individual are particularly relevant. How well do you know yourself? How close is your idea of yourself to reality, and how close is reality to the person you would like to be? The challenges you will face will test your clinical knowledge and skills but most will require you to draw on resources you did not acquire in lectures or textbooks. The resources you will need to draw on have been developed over the course of your life and include your *character, personality or self*, all of which underpin your behaviours and how you respond to and interact with other people. In the context of developing good medical practice, as well as understanding the impact of your personality on interactions, it is also important to monitor your internal states: emotions, attitudes and response to external stimuli.

This chapter provides an introduction to different ways that researchers and practitioners look at developing more self insight and understanding. After reading this chapter you will be able to:

- use a range of tools and concepts to develop self-insight, understanding of yourself and others and more mindful practice;
- recognise issues and situations that you find challenging and identify strategies to cope with these;
- identify areas for development and change.

Case study 3.1: A challenging situation?

You are an F2 on a surgical rotation and have just come on duty. The registrar is busy and has asked you to go and examine Mike who is just recovering from emergency surgery after a serious road traffic accident. Mike is 18 years old and was joy riding with a friend, Steve, through a residential area. While being pursued by the police they knocked over and killed an 8-year-old girl, then hit a lamppost at high speed. In the crash, Mike and Steve were both badly injured but later Steve was pronounced dead at the scene. Mike is unlikely to regain any function or feeling below the waist. He will need a significant degree of rehabilitation and support to adapt to his new circumstances. Mike's parents are both with him. You know that you will also need to answer any questions he or his parents might have.

ACTIVITY 3.1 A CHALLENGING SITUATION?

You are about to go and speak to Mike. Re-read these three competencies from the list above:

- Acts with empathy, honesty and sensitivity in a non-confrontational manner.
- Respects and supports the privacy and dignity of patients.
- Has a non-judgemental approach.

Being honest with yourself, would you find it challenging to display these competencies?
Which would you find most challenging and why?
Is this due to your prior experiences?
What information, advice or support might you need before (or after) going to talk with Mike and his parents, and how would you ensure this?

Who do you think you are?

People have been fascinated with the idea of systems that will reveal their personalities for centuries. A Google search for *personality test* receives nearly nine million hits. Many of these methods, such as palmistry, astrology and phrenology have been closely linked with ways to predict character and associated behaviours. The popularity of personality testing continues unabated, from the 'recreational' end of the scale, commonly seen in questionnaires in magazines and on the web, to serious psychological profiling systems used in recruitment, leadership training and professional development. You may

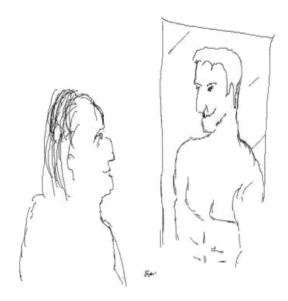

Figure 3.1 Who do you think you are?

already have taken part in some kind of personality assessment either before or during your undergraduate training. If this is the case, try to recall how the process felt, how effective you thought it was at the time, and if it proved to be of any lasting value to you.

Two of the most widely-used and generally reliable personality indicators are the Myers Briggs Personality Type Indicator (MBTI) and the NEO Personality Inventory (NEO PI-R).

Myers Briggs Personality Type Indicator (MBTI)

The MBTI is used worldwide across all types of organisations, and though it is a methodology for determining an individual's personality type *preference*, it is most frequently used for organisational purposes such as diagnosing organisational issues, team building, and leadership development. Individuals may find it helpful as part of a programme of counselling, career development or planning or improving interpersonal and communication skills

The MBTI is an extensive questionnaire consisting entirely of *forced choices* between two possible answers. The theory is based on identifying patterns which are consistent with Jung's Psychological Types. When completed, a participant receives a *personality inventory* which gives them a four letter code (e.g. ISTJ, ENFP) indicating their personality preferences out of a possible 16 Personality Types. The different type preferences indicate different ways of processing information and making decisions. They describe different approaches to working, learning styles, way of managing, leading, and coaching as well as communication and relational style. They also give an indication as to how people cope under stress. The MBTI is not a clinical inventory. All the types are healthy, with their own strengths and weaknesses. No preferences are better or worse than others, just different.

Jung's type preferences

Jung considered that people had innate preferences for four personality opposites:

- *Extraversion or Introversion* (E or I) – whether people draw their emotional energy and stimulation from the external world and other people, or the internal world of thoughts, concepts and ideas. Introverts predominate in the professions such as medicine and law, also (perhaps surprisingly) in politics.

- *Sensing or Intuition* (S or N) – whether people draw their conclusions about external stimuli through the data received via their five senses, or the 'facts' as they see them, or whether they would prefer to reflect on the external evidence and draw conclusions based on their own interpretation.

- *Thinking or Feeling* (T or F) – whether a person perceives him/herself as making decisions based on the objective evidence or 'truth', or based on the application of personal values to the issue. Thinking people predominate in medicine and law, while Feeling people are more numerous in counselling and many of the helping professions.

- *Judgement or Perceiving* (J or P) – how people tend to make decisions. A Judging person likes decisions and to be scheduled and ordered, expecting the same of others, whereas a Perceiving person may leave a decision until the last moment, liking a spontaneous approach to life and work.

While the MBTI can reveal a person's type preference with some degree of accuracy, it does not predict behaviours because they are subject to many other competing factors. It cannot account for the influence of culture and upbringing and is less useful in predicting what people will do than in helping to understand why and how they do things a certain way.

ACTIVITY 3.2 APPLYING MYERS BRIGGS IN PRACTICE

Find someone you know who has done the MBTI. Ask them what their Personality Type is according to their results. Don't discuss their results with them.

Go to www.capt.org/mbti-assessment/type-descriptions.htm

Do you think the Personality Type accurately reflects the person you know?

You can discuss the results with the person you know now if you wish.

The NEO Personality Inventory (NEO PI-R)

The NEO PI-R is widely used in the context of clinical, counselling, educational and training environments. It is based on the Five-Factor (or 'Big 5' personality types) model and is designed to provide a general description of normal personality.

NEO PI-R items and materials are designed to be easily read and understood. The five domains (factors) measured by the NEO PI-R provide a general description of personality, while the facet scales allow more detailed analysis. These five factors and their facet scales include:

- *neuroticism* (anxiety, hostility, depression, self-consciousness, impulsiveness, vulnerability);

- *extraversion* (warmth, gregariousness, assertiveness, activity, excitement-seeking, positive emotions);

- *openness to experience* (fantasy, aesthetics, feelings, actions, ideas, values);

- *agreeableness* (trust, modesty, compliance, altruism, straightforwardness, tender-mindedness);

- *conscientiousness* (competence, self-discipline, achievement-striving, dutifulness, order, deliberation).

So what?

In medicine and healthcare, like any field of professional endeavour, the whole range of personality types will be encountered. It used to be thought that certain personality types suited particular specialties. However a review of the evidence of a link between personality type and specialty choice (which included studies on the MBTI as well as on five-factor model measures of personality) concluded the following:

> There is more variation in personality traits within medical specialties than between them. Accordingly, one must conclude that all personality types appear in all specialties, and then assert that more than one specialty fits the personality of any particular medical student.
>
> (Borges and Savickas, 2002)

In addition there is evidence that personality types change over time.

So you may wonder why bother? If the assessments are used to help increase your own self-knowledge and exploration of your own motives of your behaviours, they can prove invaluable.

Is it a matter of style?

Table 3.1 shows 'target styles' within the three centre columns. On the horizontal axis there are five distinct styles, and on the vertical six domains in which those styles may be observed. Doctors and other health professionals whose behaviours are in the middle columns tend to be more adept at teamwork, relationships with patients and the public, interprofessional working and self-care (see Chapters 7 and 13 for more on this). It is extremely important to note that with increasing experience and confidence doctors learn to locate themselves at the point on the *three* centre columns that is most appropriate to the immediate context.

Table 3.1 Five distinct behavioural styles for dealing with people

	(1) Submissive	(2) Caring	(3) Collaborative	(4) Compelling	(5) Aggressive
Degree of Assertiveness	No assertiveness	Low assertiveness	Mid assertiveness	High assertiveness	Off the scale into intimidation
How You Come Across	Disinterested, passive, shy or not opinionated	Interested, caring and supportive	Collaborative and a team player, willing to both give and take	Persuasive and assertive, yet not running over others	Aggressive and overbearing
Behavioural Emphasis	Avoid conflict, don't rock the boat	Show empathy and understanding to others	An equal emphasis on personal needs and the needs of others	Emphasis on personal needs and asserting personal views	Run over people to get your way
Involvement of Others	No involvement ('Whatever you want is fine with me')	High involvement	Mid involvement	Low involvement	No involvement ('My way or the highway')
Communication Style	No openness in communication	Asking questions, clarifying, summarising, and empathising (emphasis on trying to understand others)	Equal mixture of asking questions and selling your viewpoint	Persuading, selling and showing enthusiasm for your viewpoint (emphasis on trying to be understood by others)	One-way communication; little or not listening
Effect on Others	No respect; take you for granted; low morale	Willingness to respond honestly	Desire to work together; teamwork	Willing to respond positively if ideas are good	Compliance, resentment, feeling defeated; anger

Source: Collegiate Project Services (2006), reproduced with kind permission from the authors.

As an example, if as an F1 you are the only doctor on scene at an emergency, you will need to be more compelling (4) than caring (2) so that you can galvanise those around you into action. On the other hand, if one of your F1 colleagues asks to meet you for coffee after his first week on A & E to discuss some problems, perhaps he might be expecting more (2) and less (4).

Self-knowledge and the practice of medicine

ACTIVITY 3.3 YOUR VISION AND THE REALITY

Think back to when you started at medical school.

- What did you imagine it would be like when you became a doctor?
- Did you imagine yourself on the wards?
- If you did, what did the patients do in that vision?
- How did you view yourself interacting with patients and with colleagues?

From the perspective of professional and organisational development, as well as satisfying individual curiosity, gaining deeper insight into your personality and how it may manifest itself is very helpful. Leadership development, team building and management programmes routinely incorporate personality assessments, and once carried out with participants they become a point of reference against which they can monitor their personal growth and professional development. This in turn suggests a strong link between self-knowledge and improved performance, one of the fundamental concepts underpinning the theory of *Emotional Intelligence* (Goleman, 1998). Many professionals are intelligent and effective in their technical field, but may not have a particularly high level of emotional intelligence or EQ (as opposed to IQ), now widely considered a core component of professional and interpersonal effectiveness in the workplace. Hospitals and health systems are highly complex environments in which the EQ of the junior doctor will be tested. Making the transition from student to practitioner involves a great deal more than putting knowledge and skills acquired in training into practice in the 'real world' (see Chapter 14).

ACTIVITY 3.4 PATIENTS AS PARTNERS

With your responses to Activity 3.3 still in mind, read this extract from the General Medical Council's *Duties of a Doctor*:

> Work in partnership with patients

- Listen to patients and respond to their concerns and preferences.
- Give patients the information they want or need in a way they can understand.
- Respect patients' right to reach decisions with you about their treatment and care.
- Support patients in caring for themselves to improve and maintain their health.

Did any of these feature in your early vision?

The transition from medical student to junior doctor is a significant rite of passage, though sometimes this is downplayed. Rites of passage are, by nature, significant but stressful events marking major life changes, and in the transition to junior doctor the new graduate may fail to leave relatively little 'baggage' behind and take on much more. One thing left behind is freedom from accountability and responsibility which came with being 'just' a student. This is outweighed by the heavy expectations a new doctor feels from all sides: the medical school that trained you, the organisation that has given you a job, your friends and family, the 'profession' and regulatory bodies and weightiest of all, yourself.

Current graduates embarking on the Foundation Programme curriculum are better prepared for practice than in previous times and experience a smoother transition to clinical practice. However, Brennan et al. (2010) conclude that, while recent changes are improving the process, there is still room for improvement in the way students are prepared and supported in the early stages. The experience is still arduous and stressful, particularly in the first year (Illing et al., 2008).

Dealing with your new responsibilities, managing fairly constant uncertainty, experiencing the sudden death of patients, working in multi-professional teams, and feeling unsupported are all sources of anxiety and stress. These sources of stress, predictable and understandable as they are, are often at odds with the stereotype of the doctor as a caring professional, empathic but ultimately maintaining the objective distance of the scientist. For you, managing the role shift from student to full-time working members of a new professional community to which you have previously been given only limited access is a significant life event.

To this new environment, you as the new graduate brings all your new skills and knowledge, plus the sum of life experiences to date: parental influences, likes and dislikes, hopes and fears, personal and spiritual beliefs, aspirations and disappointments, every contributory factor in the process that has lead to this experience of a Foundation rotation in a specific organisation and specialty.

In the earliest stages of the development of the 'new' doctor, you may be overwhelmed by the sheer volume and complexity of the inputs that you can be bombarded with. Brennan et al.'s (2010) respondents were particularly graphic: one suggesting there is 'no greater challenge outside of war time', another describing the experience as 'terrifying'.

Though there is an argument that no one can be totally prepared for the radical changes they will experience in their life, when they become a junior doctor the better a person knows him or herself, then they will, in turn, *be* better prepared.

ACTIVITY 3.5 A DIFFICULT SITUATION?

You are on duty in A&E on a relatively quiet Saturday afternoon when the wife of one of the oncology consultants' presents with a suspected fracture of the radius. She is dressed for riding and says she fell off her horse. Her daughter brought her in. This is the second time in a year she has had a similar injury, and after examining her and hearing discrepancies in her story you are not convinced that it is the result of a riding accident.

Make a note of your immediate reaction to this scenario, then look at the Foundation Programme Curriculum:

www.foundationprogramme.nhs.uk/pages/home/key-documents#curriculum

Decide which of the competences apply in this case, and think through the possible course of action you would take and *why*. Try to pin down any underlying *non-clinical* reasons which may influence your decision.

The emergence of professional identity as part of the self

Figure 3.2 captures something of the complex and often competing influences which come to bear on the professional and personal formation of the junior doctor in the course of daily working life.

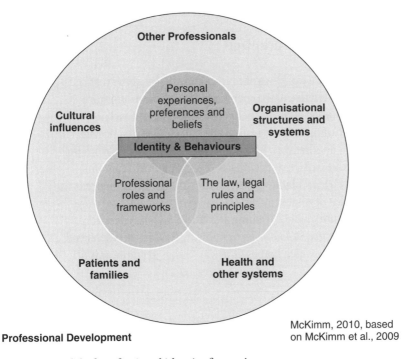

Figure 3.2 A model of professional identity formation

In developing an identity as a 'doctor', an individual faces many more challenges than those of clinical responsibilities. The three circles in the centre represent three major 'forces' at play in forming the identity and behaviours of the new professional, their intersects representing the emergent 'mix'. This identity formation is also influenced by constant and often competing inputs from the wider social, cultural and health environment, such as those represented in the diagram by patients and families, other professionals and other systems (such as the healthcare organisation, departments and specialities, social services, local authorities, the police and legal systems, primary care organisations, etc.).

Into this arrives you, the new doctor, with pre-existing behaviours and identity, and *none* of the above is static. You will develop an understanding about the profession and its boundaries. These sets of beliefs, attitudes and understanding about their roles contribute to your 'professional identity' (Lingard et al., 2003) which is framed within the context of your social identity. The final stage in the establishment of a professional identity is *integrating (doctor) into self* (Gregg and Magilvy, 2001). This involves incorporating new role behaviours and attitudes into an adjusted view of the self but as Bleakley (2006) suggests, this professional identity is also continually being (re)-constructed and altered through discourse between individuals. The more comfortable you become with your emerging role as a doctor and see this as continually evolving through interaction with other doctors, health professionals and patients, the more your professional self will develop. Consciously observing how doctors and other health professionals work and interact will provide insight into how your own personality and behaviours may need to be modified and developed.

Self-knowledge as part of your practice

It is perhaps tempting to imagine the workings of a typical hospital as some vast drama being played out, and as a relative newcomer feel as if somebody only gave you part of the script, but in fact none of the participants is an actor and each individual role is only too real. According to Good et al. (1985) 'all clinical practice has an interpretive dimension'. Put another way, junior doctors are called upon from the outset to make decisions as active participants with key roles in clinical situations, drawing on the resources they have available to them at the time the decision needs to be made. Those resources consist of what Eraut (1994) calls *propositional knowledge*: theoretical knowledge gained from medical training and study, *personal knowledge* which is gained from experience, *process knowledge* or knowing how a task is achieved and *professionally relevant know-how* which is about the way 'things get done around here'.

ACTIVITY 3.6 FIRST WEEK AS AN F1 DOCTOR

Read this doctors' account of an early experience of being an F1.

First week as an F1 doctor

Written by Dr Anirban Pal, a doctor who is just finishing his F1 year:

My first week as a foundation doctor was better than I had expected. I had a supportive team of seniors and nursing staff; they made the transition to what was my first 'real' job so much easier. Understanding that you are going from what is essentially a self-driven environment in medical school to a team-based working environment is one of the key differences and leaps you have to make when you start work this year. Remember always, that respect makes a team tick, and if you show respect you will soon become a favorite amongst equals.

Sometimes, even though it is exceedingly rare, your team may not be very supportive of you or your fledgling status – there are always other forms of support that you can access. Speak to your educational supervisor, speak to the ward sister or matron, or even a member of your family. Remember that you should never suffer in silence.

We had numerous induction sessions during the first week. These sessions, whilst mind-numbing at times, are a must. There are people there who have been working at the hospital for far longer than you have and they will have some gems of advice for the coming year. A lot of the time, they also hand out some useful kit at these sessions – I remember an antibiotic guideline card which I still carry with me. In all likelihood you'll have to fill out a number of forms and sign just as many; get used to it as your signature will become a hotly contested thing in this coming year. Dealing with the administrative machinery is one of the less pleasant experiences of the first week, but it is also absolutely necessary to ensure that the rest of your year goes smoothly. Make sure all your documents are correctly filled in and that occupational health has your correct address! You'll have to jump through a lot of hoops this coming year so get used to it and accept the suffering as part of the experience.

Back on the wards, you may feel nervous dealing with acutely ill patients in a foreign environment. Always know that you are not alone. Get help whenever you can. You'll learn best from watching expert seniors at work. Your skills at assessing patients, practical skills etc. will naturally improve during the year but always get senior help when you feel overwhelmed.

Your principal job as a houseman are the 'house-keeping jobs' (blood rounds) I spent my first days just getting comfortable with the computerised systems in use at the hospital so that I could access results, order investigations, and look at X-rays without needing any help. Also, learn the layout of your ward – where the essential equipment and crash trolley are kept, where the stationery is kept, and where the tea/coffee is kept.

Equally important during these first few weeks is to get to know your fellow foundation trainees. Be sociable and open. A good beginning will win you a lot of friends for the rest of the year. You will need all the friends you can get to swap on-calls, cover shifts, and just generally to 'discuss' the frustrations of work

What makes a good foundation trainee, my consultant told me, is not a genius but a person who is honest, reliable and trustworthy. Aim to be all of these things during this year and you will make the right impression on the right people.

(Copyright Dr Anirban Pal.
Source: NHS Medical Careers (**www.medicalcareers.nhs.uk/medical_
students/first_week_as_an_f1_doctor.aspx**). Reprinted with permission)

- Note down the hints and tips you think will be of practical help to you.
- Reflect on the impression you have of the author. Try to work out how you arrived at it, and what it is about *you* that contributed to it.

Clearly a junior doctor at the start of the Foundation Programme is likely to rely heavily on propositional knowledge and hope to build up the remaining three as quickly as possible, but unfortunately they don't lend themselves to acquisition by study alone as they are much more complex than 'book learning'. Personal knowledge, gained from experience, is limited in the early stage to that gained on placements, and much of it will be observed rather than experienced, but it also comprises intuitions and interpretations collected along the way, often outside conscious awareness. Some of these may predate the period of professional training and have their origin in a personal experience, a remark made by a significant adult or a TV series. Horsburgh et al. (2006) suggest that medical and other healthcare students have specific beliefs and opinions about the way work should be undertaken and that the process of professional socialisation and attitude, belief and value formation (professional identity) has already begun before students enter professional education.

Process knowledge concerns how a particular task is done, such as gathering relevant information, performing the procedure and making future care decisions. Process knowledge also includes reflecting on one's own mental processes.

To become more aware of one's own mental processes, listen more attentively, become flexible, and recognize bias and judgments, and thereby act with principles and compassion.

(Epstein, 1999, p835)

Professionally relevant knowledge, or the art of knowing how to get things done, is likely to be gained more rapidly by those with higher levels of emotional intelligence, since it involves not only knowing *who* one needs to know but *how* to cultivate the right relationships with them (see Chapter 18).

Epstein uses a phrase from Anaïs Nin 'We don't see things as they are, we see things as we are' (1969, p834) to emphasise that all clinical decision-making involves more than an empirical evidence-based judgement. Physician factors such as bias, emotions, prejudice, risk aversion and levels of empathy can all influence the final outcome, some more overtly than others. This should not be too surprising since doctors' backgrounds and personalities create the basis for their position in the social world, and their personal experiences and attitudes form the grounds for understanding each patient. You as the junior doctor need to practise mindfully just as much as the seasoned physician, and learn to recognise how their experiences, backgrounds and personalities have a bearing on your professional practice and your relationships with patients. Participating in case conferences, significant event analyses and clinical governance activities such as audits will all help you gain insight into how professional behaviours can impact on effective and safe medical practice and what lessons might be learned.

The Johari Window (see Figure 3.3) is a tool to better understand your interpersonal communication and relationships characteristics. It is often pictorially represented as four panes or quadrants in a window. The technique involves revealing more of the 'blind' quadrant by *asking* people about what they think of you and how they see you so you find out more about yourself as seen through others. It also involves revealing more of yourself from the 'hidden' quadrant by *telling* people more about you so that they understand you better. In this way you expand your self-insight and understanding and develop deeper relationships with others.

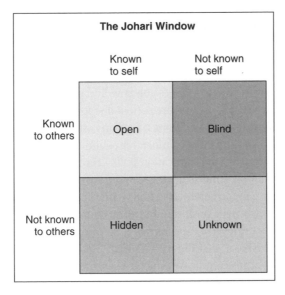

Figure 3.3 The Johari Window

ACTIVITY 3.7 ACCEPTING FEEDBACK

Think about a time when you have received feedback from a supervisor and how you felt about it? Often feedback confirms what we already know (the 'open' pane in the window), but sometimes it can be feedback that we find hard to accept (usually the 'blind' pane in the window, sometimes the 'hidden' pane). This challenging feedback is often the hardest to accept but can provide the best self-insight and understanding such as if you were unaware that your manner could be perceived as brusque or arrogant, when you thought you were being efficient and capable.

Try it for yourself at: **http://kevan.org/johari**

You will need the help of some friends who know you quite well to practise the techniques of telling and asking, you may also use this technique with your supervisor.

Self-knowledge and interacting with colleagues, patients and families

Many of the outcomes and competencies from the Foundation Programme Curriculum involve interactions with colleagues, patients and the public, and you will need to be competent in all of them. 'Mindful practice' helps you to reflect on interactions that occur in the course of your practice, giving you an opportunity to analyse what went well, what went less so, what you might do differently next time and, importantly, why you may have done or said certain things.

Interacting with colleagues in today's healthcare system calls for a high degree of interprofessional collaboration as you will read in Chapter 13. This implies a degree of responsibility to understand the world in which your colleagues practice and how it interfaces with yours, and a sense of what they need from you in order to do their job properly.

Communicating with patients is the cornerstone of good medical practice, yet mishandled communication has been the cause of more patient dissatisfaction, critical incidents, bad publicity and individual physician angst than any other single factor (see Chapters 7 and 8). Some doctors are more comfortable communicators than others. There are many ways of improving communication skills – through training, through mindfulness and self-evaluation – and all doctors can improve their skills. Knowing yourself is a good starting point in communication terms. There will always be certain people or types of people who will 'push your buttons'. Usually it is because of some memory planted well below the level of consciousness, so you don't recognise the stimuli. It could be someone who has a voice like a particularly obnoxious uncle from early childhood, or somebody whose physical characteristics resemble a long forgotten school bully. It may be an ethnic or social group that you somehow internalised negative 'messages' about at an early age.

It may, however, be none of the above. Sometimes even before the consultation, the patient has ideas about the doctor (or the health system) and is imposing his or her own meanings on the situation. All health workers are taught that every patient is an individual, but patients are not subject to professional constraints: some tend to see doctors as all the same, others mistrust the medical profession, still more have impossibly high expectations.

Self-awareness can also help the reflective practitioner realise when the *primary* problem in a bad communication does not lie with them.

Understanding yourself – going forwards

> Self-knowledge is less a matter of careful introspection than of becoming an excellent observer of oneself.
>
> (Wilson, 2009)

Developing yourself as a professional involves moving on from the idea that self-knowledge is about assessing personality, and then ascribing our actions, feelings and reactions to whatever that assessment may have revealed. Instead, the modern medical practitioner should be acquiring the technique of accurate self-monitoring on a day-to-day basis and participating in developmental activities that provide useful feedback on the non-technical skills as well as clinical procedures or management. Multi-source Feedback assessments such as TAB help provide feedback on communication and teamworking skills, but you may wish to explore other means of acquiring feedback on your interpersonal skills and qualities or the way you handled situations through peer mentoring, action learning sets or other support groups. It may be tempting to dismiss this idea as advocating self-indulgent 'navel-gazing', but in reality there is little that differentiates this practice from keeping a close eye on one's own physical health and general fitness. If, on the other hand, self-awareness is only part of a systematic approach to constantly reviewing, refining and improving one's practice, it can become part of a habitual commitment to quality.

Mindful practice offers you a template for reflective practice, gaining a deeper understanding of yourself as a developing professional, mapping progress, owning and learning from mistakes and building technical competence, presence and insight.

In conclusion

Knowing yourself better is not just an aid to better medical practice, it is a vital element in any field of endeavour. The more you understand about who you are, where you came from, the cultural and other environmental influences that formed the current you, the motivations, hopes and fears that underpin your decisions and will drive your potential, the more likely the endeavour will achieve the outcomes you seek. As with all knowledge, there will never be a time when you know it all, but the target should be day-to-day self-monitoring at the level of unconscious competence.

Chapter summary

- Personality assessments can reveal behavioural preferences which are conscious and cognitive. They cannot account for beliefs and motivations operating outside conscious awareness.

- Most people draw on more than one behavioural style according to the demands of the situation. Emotional intelligence includes being situationally aware and behaviourally adept enough to know exactly when to do so, and which style to adopt.

- The goals of mindful practice are 'To become more aware of one's own mental processes, listen more attentively, become flexible, and recognise bias and judgments, and thereby act with principles and compassion'. If these are embraced early in a medical career, they become embedded and habitual.

- Today's foundation doctors are tomorrow's clinical leaders. Leadership skills can be learned and acquired through experience, but are also founded on sound self knowledge and awareness.

GOING FURTHER

General Medical Council (2009) *Tomorrow's Doctors*. London: General Medical Council. **www.gmc-uk.org/undergraduate_education_publications. asp#1**

General Medical Council (2009) *Medical Students: Professional Behaviour and Fitness to Practise*. London: General Medical Council. **www.gmc-uk.org/undergraduate_education_publications.asp#medical**

Myers Briggs Types Inventory. **www.personalitypathways.com/MBTI_intro. html**

Swanwick, T (2005) Informal Learning in Postgraduate Medical Education: from Cognitivism to 'Culturism'. *Medical Education,* 39, 859–865

Wilson, TD (2009) Knowing me, myself and I: what psychology can contribute to self-knowledge. *Perspectives on Psychological Science,* Association for Psychological Science (8 September).

chapter 4

Planning Your Career Development
Caroline Elton

Achieving foundation competences

This chapter will help you to begin to meet the following requirements of the *Foundation Programme Curriculum* (2010):

- Understand how appraisal promotes lifelong learning and professional development including career progression (p46).
- Develop career planning skills (p64).
- Use the Foundation Programme to explore wider career options before giving detailed attention to a specific career pathway (p64, also Foundation Reference Guide 2010, 9.34).
- Adopt a pragmatic, realistic outlook to choosing a specialty (p64, also Foundation Reference Guide 2010, 9.34).
- Understand that careers can change due to ill health, disability and work–life balance issues, and the sources of support available in these circumstances (p65, also Foundation Reference Guide 2010, 9.34).
- Use the e-portfolio as the basis for career discussions (p65).

Chapter overview

This chapter sets out a framework for career planning, both in the short and the longer term. The importance of adopting a structured approach to career planning is discussed and a four-stage model (self-assessment, option exploration, decision-making and plan implementation) is described in some detail. This chapter explains the links between career planning and educational appraisal and sources of support for more complex career difficulties are outlined.

After reading this chapter you will be able to:

- describe the four-stage model of career planning;
- identify appropriate career resources to help you with each of the four stages;
- use your e-portfolio as an essential component of career planning;
- understand the role of educational appraisal, in both the short and the longer term.

Career planning in the context of Modernising Medical Careers (MMC)

Since the introduction of the Modernising Medical Careers reforms in August 2005, the issue of careers advice has gained greater prominence within medical education. Under the new MMC training structure, trainees have to make major career decisions about specialty choice 18 months after finishing their undegraduate training. Prior to the introduction of MMC, many trainees had not decided on their final specialty at this point in their career (Goldacre et al., 2004, 2010). Recognising that trainees now have to make significant career decisions at an earlier stage of their postgraduate training, the independent enquiry into the MMC reforms recommended that more attention needed to be given to the issue of careers support, from medical school onwards (Tooke, 2008).

The importance of a shared framework

A large-scale study of work-based career discussions (i.e. discussions taking place between a supervisor and a supervisee) reported that if both parties had a shared framework of how the discussion should be structured, the supervisee found the discussion to be more useful (Hirsh et al., 2001). This makes intuitive sense because if neither party know what the discussion should be focusing on, it is more likely to become a somewhat aimless 'chat'.

Using the four-stage model

The framework that is commonly used in higher education careers suport, both generally, and within medical education, is the four-stage model.

The four stages are as follows:

1 Self-assessment.

2 Career exploration.

3 Decision-making.

4 Plan implementation.

The Association of American Medical Colleges' online career planning resource (Careers in Medicine) on which the UK's national medical careers website (**www. medicalcareers.nhs.uk**) is based, both use this structure.

Stage 1: Self-assessment

Just as good clinical diagnosis depends upon taking a thorough patient history, good career decision-making rests on thorough self-assessment. There are numerous potential aspects that you could consider as part of the self-assessment stage but (as a bare minimum) you need to be clear about your core work values, interests, key skills, and potential stressors. Self-assessment exercises are available on the national medical careers website (**www.medicalcareers.nhs.uk**). Other approaches to self-assesssment are listed on the bottom of the Medicine on Track (MOT) career planning form (see Activity 4.1).

Recent research (e.g. the 2008 BMA study on professional values) has shown that the majority of doctors believe that a career in medicine should not preclude having an acceptable work–life balance. So, when you are reviewing your core work values as part of the self-assessment stage, you need to consider the relationship that you want between your professional life and your personal life. For example, specialties differ significantly in their out-of-hours commitments, both during specialty training and as a consultant, so you need to factor in the sort of work–life balance that is acceptable to you.

Stage 2: Career exploration

There are two important points to make about Stage 2. First, career exploration should not be undertaken in a vacuum: the particular issues you need to explore in this stage relate to what you have found out about yourself in the previous self-assessment stage. In other words, you need to 'personalise' the career exploration stage, going beyond all the basic information including training routes or further professional exams.

Second, you should keep your mind open during your foundation training about career options that might suit you. Two BMA follow-up studies of a cohort that graduated from medical school in 2006 reported that half of the doctors changed their career intentions during their first foundation year (British Medical Association, 2008) and nearly the same proportion changed in their second foundation year (British Medical Association, 2009a).

Some of you may be interested in specialties that you weren't able to work in during your foundation training. This may be because you were not successful in obtaining a foundation rotation that included that particular specialty, or because foundation placements in that specialty were not on offer in any rotation. In this situation, you can apply for a short 'taster' experience in their specialty of interest. The Foundation Programme Reference Guide (UK Foundation Programme Office, 2010) gives clear advice about setting up a taster placement. On return from your taster, you will find it extremely helpful to set up a 'de-briefing' meeting with your educational or clinical supervisor in order to discuss the implications of the taster for your longer-term career plans.

Stage 3: Decision-making

As with Stage 2, there are two important points to make about how you should approach Stage 3. First, there is a need for flexibility in your decision-making. When working with junior doctors, I link this assertion to the psychological literature that suggests that despite popular stereotypes to the contrary, there is actually more variation in personality traits *within* specialties than *between* them (Borges and Savickas, 2002). Borges et al. (2004) go on to argue that early on in their medical training, individuals should be disabused of the notion that for each person there is only one specialty that would suit them. In fact there are over 60 different specialties to choose from and I frequently challenge foundation trainees by asking them how they know that they wouldn't like a particular specialty if they know absolutely nothing about it.

The second point is that if you don't feel ready to make a career decision about specialty choice at the appropriate time in your second foundation year, you should give serious consideration to applying for a temporary post in the interim, to help you decide. Whilst you can't delay the decision-making indefinitely, as long as you can show how you have used the interim post to help you make longer-term career decisions about specialty choice (and also how you have enhanced your CV during the year), it should not seriously disadvantage you the following year.

Stage 4: Plan implentation

Given the demanding nature of medical practice, it is tempting to leave the task of preparing your job application to the last minute. This is very understandable, but is not a strategy that is designed to maximise success.

Instead, you need to give serious consideration and thought to the final stage – plan implementation. To start with, you should keep abreast of the timetable for specialty recruitment. The easiest way to do this is to check the relevant websites regularly. As a bare miniumum I would suggest the national medical careers website (**www.medicalcareers.nhs.uk**), the MMC website (**www.mmc.nhs.uk**) and the websites of any deaneries to which you are intending to apply.

The whole application process is also linked to the person specification for that specialty, which in turn has been derived from the GMC's *Good Medical Practice* framework. You can download the previous year's person specification from the MMC website (**www.mmc.nhs.uk**), and well in advance of the recruitment process going live, you should have gone through your portfolio with a fine toothcomb and identified examples that you could write about (or discuss at the interview) that give clear evidence of each competence listed on the person specification.

Increasingly, specialties are moving away from relying solely on CV-based interviews, and are using new approaches such as machine-marked tests, group interviews and observed consultations with simulated patients. However, when these new approaches to recruitment and selection are being used (such as in the national GP recruitment model), detailed information is given to applicants in advance, to help them prepare. This is why it is vital to keep checking the relevant websites suggested above so you are not taken by surprise.

Links between career support and educational appraisal

In 2003, a study of medical students and junior doctors found that the most frequent source of careers support was senior clinicians, rather than careers professionals

(Jackson et al., 2003). Although in 2003 most medical schools and deaneries had only rudimentary careers services (whereas now there are designated careers advisers in all medical schools and deaneries), guidelines for both the Foundation Programme (Foundation Programme Reference Guide, 2010) and for Post-Foundation (The Gold Guide to Specialty Training – NHS, 2010) state that careers support should be provided in the context of regular educational appraisal discussions with educational supervisors.

In other words, the time and place for reviewing your career plans is during your regular appraisal meeting with your educational supervisor. Prior to your scheduled educational appraisal meeting you might want to complete Activity 4.1, which will help you to approach the task of career planning in a systematic manner.

ACTIVITY 4.1 MEDICINE ON TRACK

Download a copy of the Medicine on Track (MOT) career planning form available on the Foundation Programme website: **www.foundationprogramme.nhs.uk/pages/ trainers/sharing-best-practice#MOT** (careers planning form for trainees).

The form is structured according to the four-stage framework; self-assessment; career exploration; decision-making; plan implementation.

Print out the form and, starting with Stage 1, work your way through it. If you realise that you need to spend more time on Stage 1, then suggestions for suitable resources to help you with self-assessment are given at the bottom of the second page of the form.

Bring the MOT form to your next educational appraisal session. You don't need to have completed it – just fill it out as far as you can.

Prior to the appraisal session review the form and note down any summary points about how your career plans are progressing.

The role of the e-portfolio

All foundation doctors have to maintain an e-portfolio and use it to support their educational and professional development, including career planning. Post-Foundation specialty trainees in all specialties also have to maintain a portfolio, although some specialties have not yet transferrred to electronic versions.

The e-portfolio provides a structured record of the foundation doctor's assessments, achievements and other evidence demonstrating that they have completed key outcomes specified by the GMC. It should be used as part of all educational appraisal discussions with your educational supervisor, and will assist you in identifying key educational outcomes for each placement. Your educational supervisor will also use it when completing your final end of placement assessment.

The purpose of the e-portofolio is not merely to serve as a record of progress, but also to help you with the task of reflection. Case study 4.1 describes a situation in which a trainee choses a specialty (oncology) which he found acutely psychologically demanding, probably linked to the earlier death of his father from cancer. Perhaps if he had maintained a portfolio in medical school (as some schools now require), he would have reflected at that time on his response to patients with cancer and gained some insight that despite his interest in the subject, he might have difficulties if he chose to specialise in oncology.

Case study 4.1: Choosing your specialty, the importance of reflective portfolios

Nicholas was a trainee doctor of Chinese origin, brought up and edu-cated in the UK. Following his parents' divorce he went to live with his father. But when Nicholas was 14 his father developed cancer and within a short time period became seriously ill and died. This was a very difficult period in his (and the rest of his family's) life and as a result, Nicholas did not perform as well as expected in the latter years of his school career. He failed to get the grades for medical school, and instead studied another scientific discipline at university. Gradu-ating with a first-class degree, he then succesfully applied to medi-cal school and started his training on a graduate entry programme. On his oncology attachment in medical school there was a young Chi-nese man on the ward. When the ward round got to this patient's bed, Nicholas fainted. This had never happened before, nor was it repeated in other clinical firms. Nicholas completed medical school without any difficulty and passed his postgraduate exams, but he found it difficult to choose a specialty. After doing a locum job in oncology, he decided to opt for specialty training in that field. Despite not having previ-ously experienced periods of anxiety or depression, within weeks of starting his oncology training he became acutely anxious. His new job also involved a long car journey and during this period he was involved in two minor car accidents, both of which were his fault. Yet he had never had a car accident before. After discussion with his supervisor and the involvement of Occupational Health, Nicholas was advised to take some sick-leave. Nicholas also consulted the deanery career counselling service and, through discussions with the deanery careers adviser, began to see that his choice of speciality had placed a con-siderable emotional load on him, due to the distress his father's death had caused him years earlier. What was particularly striking was the indication that he might find working in oncology difficult from his dramatic response at the Chinese patient's bedside years earlier at medical school.

SMART objectives

At the end of each educational appraisal, you should agree some educational objectives on which you will concentrate between this appraisal and the next. These objectives might relate to a specific clinical issue, or they might relate directly to a career planning issue (e.g. organising a taster to explore whether or not you might be suited to a particular specialty).

Whether the task is directly or indirectly related to career planning, it can be helpful to formulate it using the SMART acronoym (see Box 4.1).

Box 4.1 SMART Objectives

Specific   Do you know exactly what the task is that you have agreed to complete?
Measurable   Do you know how you will measure whether or not you have
              completed this task?
Achievable   Will you be able to complete this task?
Relevant*   Is this task relevant to your broader aims?
Time-bound   Have you agreed a time-frame for completing this task?

* Some authors use 'Realistic' instead of 'Relevant'. I recommend the latter, as 'Realistic'
  overlaps with Achievable. And the relevancy question is key to effective objective setting.

To give you a sense of how SMART planning works, setting an objective such as 'Finding out more about different specialties I could apply for' doesn't pass the SMART test. As an objective it is insufficiently specific, measurable, or time-bound. In contrast an objective such as 'Completing a taster in Pathology within the next three months in order to decide whether I am going to apply for that specialty' fits all the SMART criteria.

The underlying psychology is really quite simple: if you know exactly *what* it is that you should be doing, *how* you will know when you have completed it, that it is *possible* to get it done, that it has a *purpose* and what your *deadline* is – you are more likely to get on and get the task done. Activity 4.2 gives you an opportunity to try this out by setting a SMART career planning objective.

ACTIVITY 4.2 SETTING SMART OBJECTIVES

The SMART acronym can be used to help you with setting educational objectives. Focusing on educational objectives related to developing your career plans, identify one specific task that you are going to complete once you have finished this chapter and that will you help you further your career plans. Then, formulate this task as a 'SMART' objective (i.e. making sure that it is **S**pecific, **M**easurable, **A**chievable, **R**elevant (and/or **R**ealistic) and **T**ime-bound).

Appraisal in the longer term

Regular appraisals are a key component of educational supervision, from the Foundation Programme onwards. You will continue having regular educational appraisals with your educational supervisor when you are a specialty or vocational trainee, and furthermore you will also have annual appraisals when you have completed your specialty/General Practice training. Once you are on the GP or Specialist Register, your annual appraisal will form a central component of your periodic revalidation with the GMC. Further details of the GMC's framework for appraisal and its link to revalidation are available on the GMC website (**www.gmc-uk.org**). Perhaps the key point to take on board is that reflective practice, appraisals, objective setting and career planning will continue throughout the whole of your medical career.

Trainees with complex career needs

For the majority of trainees, formal career discussions linked to educational appraisals combined with more informal discussions with other senior clinicians provide sufficient careers' support. But some trainees have more complex needs and in this situation professional careers support can be helpful. Trainees seeking one-to-one career counselling from the deanery careers service that I head up typically come for the following sorts of reasons: an inability to decide on the next step; wanting to explore options outside of clinical practice, struggling with a physical or mental health issue and repeated failure of exams. A full list of deanery-based careers advisers is given on the Foundation Programme website (**www.foundationprogramme. nhs.uk**).

Chapter summary

This chapter has:

- outlined a structured approach to career planning;

- explained how career planning discussions take place in the context of regular educational appraisal meetings;

- provided suggestions on how to get the most from your appraisal discussions by preparing in advance, using your e-portfolio and setting SMART objectives.

GOING FURTHER

When you are at the 'Career Exploration' stage, you can use the specialty pages of the national medical careers website **www.medicalcareers.nhs.uk** to read about some of the smaller specialties that you might know very little about.

Look on your deanery website, or the BMJ Careers website and see if there is a forthcoming Careers Fair. These events provide an opportunity to learn about many different career options, and also to receive help with CVs, application forms and interview preparation.

When you are preparing for a forthcoming interview, look at the DVD *Selection Centres for Speciality Training* produced by the South West Peninsula Deanery in conjunction with the Association of Graduate Careers Advisory Services (AGCAS). The DVD gives in-depth coverage of interview and assessment processes and should be available through your Trust library or foundation school. Alternatively, contact **www.agcas.org.uk/agcas_resources.**

part 2

Putting the Patient First and Improving Services

chapter 5

Clinical Governance and Quality Improvement

Sue Lister

Achieving foundation competences

This chapter will help you to begin to meet the following requirements of the *Foundation Programme Curriculum* (2010).

Outcome 7 Patient safety within clinical governance

Demonstrates a clear commitment to maintaining patient safety and delivering high-quality reliable care. Understand that clinical governance is the overarching framework that unites a range of quality improvement activities to safeguard standards and facilitate improvements in clinical services.

7.1 Treats the patient as the centre of care

- Listens actively and enables patients to express concerns and preferences, ask questions and make personal choices.
- Respects the right to autonomy and confidentiality.
- Recognises the patient's confidence and competence to self-care and need for support, notably when an acute problem is superimposed on a chronic illness.
- Seeks advice promptly when unable to answer a patient's query or concerns.
- Respects the patient's right to refuse treatment or take part in research.
- Considers care pathways and the process of care from the patient's perspective.
- Describes common reactions of patients, family and clinical staff to error.
- Places the needs of patients above own convenience without compromising the safety of self or others.

7.4 Understands the principles of quality and safety improvement

- Demonstrates knowledge of how and when to report adverse events and 'near misses' to local and, where appropriate, national reporting systems.
- Describes opportunities for improving the reliability of care following adverse events or 'near misses'.
- Describes root cause analysis.

Knowledge

- Definition of clinical governance and its various components.
- The theoretical and policy frameworks for clinical governance.
- The contribution of clinical governance to the monitoring and continuous improvement of the quality of healthcare.

Chapter overview

This chapter aims to consider how government policy drives the need to improve services and monitoring of how we provide care and offers a range of tools and models which you can use to maintain and improve health service quality. The underpinning focus of service improvement is understanding care from the patient/service-user perspective. Various concepts, tools and models will be used to show how to monitor care provision, including: the audit cycle, clinical governance, risk management, root cause analysis and critical incidence reporting. We will look at the role of protocols, checklists and guidelines in maintaining quality care through best practice. The overriding approach is how to improve services by focusing on processes.

After reading this chapter you will be able to:

• discuss the major policy drivers underpinning service improvement;
• identify areas of risk and potential innovation in your own healthcare context;
• apply tools and models to maintaining a quality healthcare service.

Policy drivers

In the 1990s, a number of major scandals rocked the NHS which are often quoted as the reason for the introduction of policies to monitor and drive improvement in healthcare provision:

• Between February and April of 1991 the child health nurse Beverly Allitt killed 13 of her patients; she is thought to have *Munchausen Syndrome* and was given a 30-year life sentence.

• Throughout the early 1990s information started to leak out about the much higher than average number of children dying while undergoing heart surgery at the Bristol Royal Infirmary, resulting in surgeons being struck off the medical register, and the re-organisation of the accountability for quality within hospital structures.

• In 1998 GP Harold Shipman was arrested for the murder of 15 of his patients. He is actually thought to have murdered more than 150 people and is Britain's most prolific mass murderer. He committed suicide in prison.

However, the dates of the introduction of the initial policies to monitor the quality of the provision of healthcare shows that the scandals ran concurrent to a change in government thinking about the need to scrutinise how healthcare was provided. A number of government White Papers (*Promoting Better Health*, 1990; *Medical Audit in the Family Practitioner Services*, 1990; *Working for Patients: Medical Audit*, 1991; *Audit Guidelines for Health Promotion Banding*, 1993) introduced medical (later to become known as 'clinical') audit into the NHS, initially in general practice. By 1997 the Patient's Charter had been published, setting out the rights and standards that patients could expect from the NHS. The first White Paper on health from first 'New Labour' government (*A First Class Service – Quality in the New NHS*, 1998) introduced clinical governance.

It can be said with confidence that the scandals strengthened government arguments for the need for monitoring the healthcare we provide – but they were not the drivers for the introduction of these policies. Politically, the 1990s was the era of questioning the quality of many public services along with their value for money. It was no longer adequate for us, as health professionals, to just assert we were good at what we did because it was clear that while some of our personal and professional quality standards were high, these were not translated into the way in which services were delivered.

In 2003 the Department of Health (DH) introduced the Knowledge and Skills Framework (KSF), replacing this initial guidance document in 2004 with the publication which presented the KSF as the career and payment strand of the Agenda for Change (Agenda for Change is the collective agreement reached between the DH and the NHS unions relating to the way NHS reforms would be implemented), thus making it an essential part of the management structure of the NHS (*The NHS Knowledge and Skills Framework and the Development Review Process*, 2004). The KSF dimensions also recognised service improvement as fundamental to the running of the NHS; Core Dimension 4 is 'Service Improvement' which underpins Core Dimension 5, which is 'Quality'.

The difference between quality and service improvement, as laid out within the KSFs, is that while quality is considered to be focused on maintaining the quality of one's own work and professional standards of clinical quality, service improvement should include:

1 Making changes within our own practice and offering suggestions for improving services.
2 Interpreting and applying suggestions, recommendations and directives to improve services.
3 Working in partnership with others to develop, take forward and evaluate direction, policies and strategies.

(DH, 2004)

The DH documents quite clearly perceive service improvement as being more about the organisational systems in which we undertake our clinical/professional activities as well as putting these activities within the wider team setting. KSF Core Dimension 4, Service Improvement, forces us to tackle the quality of care we provide from a wider perspective than just our own clinical competence.

The DH has also produced the National Service Frameworks (NSF) for particular health conditions. There are NSFs for children, diabetes, care of older people, mental health – all setting specific standards, guidance and key interventions. All health professionals now need knowledge of the NSF that is applicable to their area of work. The Department of Health provides downloadable and browsable versions of the NSFs at **www.dh.gov.uk**.

Regardless of changes in government and the possible introduction of new terminology applied to quality, the constant need to improve the quality of care we provide and the service in which we deliver them will not and should not go away.

Patient focus

Patients, service users and carers will not usually recognise a demarcation between quality and service improvement. To patients it is *all* about the quality of their care; whether it is clinical negligence, the lack of optimal care, inexplicable time delays, cleanliness (or the lack of it) or whether you treat patients with respect and dignity. In fact patients are less likely to complain about clinical competence than any of the other behaviours or actions imposed on them, because they make an assumption of clinical proficiency – people wouldn't go to the doctors if they thought doctors were dangerous. Most of the population does not have enough knowledge of medical science to challenge our clinical expertise, but they do know when we are rude, when the ward is dirty, when car parks are overcrowded and expensive, and when they are left alone for long periods of time.

Most of us take up caring professions within health and social care in order to do good, to make a difference, certainly to do the job well and most people do not go to work each day with the intention of doing harm or even of doing our job badly. However, in spite of our best intentions, patients are still left dissatisfied.

We need to understand the care we provide from the patients' perspective. There are many ways we can do this, but the vast majority of us have experienced healthcare directly, either ourselves or through a relative. A revealing discussion with colleagues about what you have experienced 'on the other side' of healthcare provision can help you remember what it feels like to be a patient. However we provide care, we must never lose sight of the patient, including enabling the patient to be central to all decisions that impact on them. We must hold on to the mantra that for the patient there should be 'nothing about me, without me' (Delbanco et al., 2001).

ACTIVITY 5.1 PATIENT CENTRED CARE

Go to **www.denisesilber.com/files/berwickyalemedicalschoolgraduationaddress-may10.pdf** and read the Yale Medical School Graduation Address, made by Donald Berwick in 2010.

Consider other ways of maintaining a focus on how it feels to be a patient.

In addition to our own reflections, we need to have a model for providing care that gives us a way of considering whether we are achieving a balanced measure of the care provided. Nelson et al.'s (1996, p21) model in Figure 5.1 provides a number of essential issues to focus on.

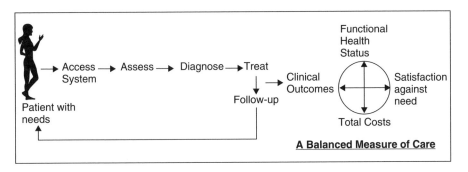

Figure 5.1 A model for providing care

Source: Nelson et al., 1996, p21

First, there is the 'patient with needs' – we don't choose our clients in the way that manufacturing and commerce can target an audience; for example, Jaguar was owned by Ford, but the Ford KA was never aimed at the same clientele as a Jaguar XJS. We have patients with needs that arrive needing our attention. Whether needing elective or emergency care, our patients come as they are, we cannot select. They have needs and they are vulnerable.

Case study 5.1: Can you put this gown on please?

When I had been qualified a few years, I asked a man in his early thirties to change so I could X-ray his lumbar spine. From the top of a heap of clean gowns I collected a folded, then ubiquitous, white gown and showing him into a cubicle, I handed it to him saying,

> 'Please take everything off except your underpants and put this on so it's fastened down the back … when you are ready come out through that door.'

I smiled pleasantly and left him to change but he didn't reappear. He was a fit man with back pain but no obvious mobility problems so I hadn't expect him to take long. After a while I knocked on the door and asked if he was OK, to which there was an affirmative grunt. I reiterated,

> 'Put the gown on so it's fastened down the back and come out when you are ready.'

He still didn't come out so I knocked on the door, opened it slightly and looked in asking,

> 'Is everything OK?'

He was in his underpants looking confused at the 'gown' and muttered,

'I don't know how to put it on.'

This was when I realised he wasn't holding a gown – I'd given him a pillowcase. I rapidly replaced it with a gown and laughed with my colleagues in the staff room about how he must surely have known it was a pillowcase so why didn't he say – one of them commented,

'Patients leave their brains in the car park.'

On reflection, I couldn't help wondering how frightened you had to be to not mention the fact it was a pillowcase. After all I was in charge, I was probably being bossy and officious, I was a clearly a highly trained professional and I must have known what I was doing. The young man was in a strange place, with that hospital smell and odd disconcerting equipment. He was probably frightened about what we might find was wrong with his back and was well and truly out of his comfort zone. In no other circumstances would this young man have sat in a cubicle for over 15 minutes trying to work out how to wear a pillowcase, open at the back or not. I now find it hard to think about this without wanting to cry – what had we done to this man to paralyse his brain and his ability to rationalise or question my instructions? From then on my behaviour changed, I was less officious and certainly more sympathetic and understanding of a patient's confusion and needs.

The next part of the model for providing care is the bit we actually impact on – the things we do. It is essential we focus on how the patients (with needs) access our service and then how we carry out the cycles of assessment, diagnosis, treatment and follow-up. This is the bit *we* do, these are the only things *we* can change to provide better, safer care.

Traditionally we have measured our activities by 'clinical outcomes' and 'total cost' but this is unbalanced. Clinical outcomes and cost need to be measured with 'functional health status' and 'satisfaction against need' or the measure isn't complete.

The young man, whose lumbar spine I X-rayed, had a good clinical outcome. The cost slightly increased because I wasted time waiting for him change, but this was insignificant – so on our traditional measures, his interaction with the X-ray department was a success. However, he can't have been satisfied, he felt humiliated and was terrified. This could impact on his functional health status because he will be *very* reluctant to return and might avoid a procedure that could give an early diagnosis to a future condition. We didn't provide a balanced measure of care.

Audit cycle, setting standards of care

Audit as defined by the DH in 1989 is:

> The systematic critical analysis of the quality of care, including procedures used for the diagnosis and treatment, the use of resources, and the resulting outcome on quality of life for the patient.

However, the fundamental aim of audit is looking at how you care for patients and seeing if it can be done better. There are a variety of versions of the audit cycle. The most basic one asks three questions:

- What *should* we be doing?
- What *are* we doing?
- What *changes* can we make?

However, it is much clearer if it is spelt out in a little more detail. The first thing to do is decide what to audit in terms of structure, process and outcomes. This decision may not be an actual part of the cycle but if it isn't clearly identified, then this step might not be acknowledged. There is a tendency for audit to default to outcomes. For example, are the feet of the patients with diabetes, that I see in the diabetes clinic, well looked after and they haven't developed gangrene? There may, however, be patients who are not attending the clinic regularly because the appointment system isn't working, or maybe there is no regular process for checking the state of people's feet – it only happens if they mention it. Therefore you have to consider whether you need to audit the structure or the process before you look at the outcome.

> *Structure* is what is physically needed to do the job, the appropriately trained staff – the equipment – the system.
> The *Process* is what you do – the implementation of protocols and agreed practices
> *Intermediate Outcome* is what we want to achieve now.
> The *Outcome* is what we ultimately achieve.
>
> (Donabedian, 1988)

The reason for the differentiation between 'Intermediate Outcome' and 'Outcome' is, for example, we may want to reduce morbidity and mortality due to smoking but that could only be measured on a national scale, through epidemiological studies – this is the outcome we ultimately want to achieve. At local level, we can measure if the number of smokers in a specific area/or registered with a general practice has reduced, this is an intermediate outcome (see Chapter 16 for more on audit and evidence-based practice).

The audit cycle (see Figure 5.2) provides a structured way of ensuring that all steps in the process are addressed. We will use the example of the state of the feet of the patients with diabetes to explain how this might work in practice.

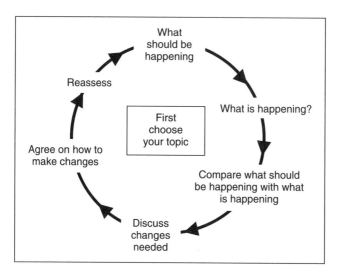

Figure 5.2 The audit cycle

Source: Lister, 1996, p6

- *Choose your topic*:

    Are we monitoring the feet of patients with diabetes?

- *What should be happening?*: this is evidence based from protocols or literature reviews. From this you can define the criterion, a specific element of care or activity that can be measured.

    Patients with diabetes should have their peripheral foot pulses monitored regularly, at least annually.

- *What is happening?*: this is the data collection – however, a pitfall of audit is to start the data collection without being specific. It is essential that a Standard is set – the actual number, count or percentage applied to a criterion.

    90% of the patients with diabetes registered at a specific general practice have had their peripheral foot pulses monitored in the last 12 months.

- *Discuss the changes needed*: this is where the activity has to become multidisciplinary. Change has to be managed and it is essential that the team that has to make the changes are involved. This is the point where many audits fail and become an audit semi-circle – an interesting data collection with no action is not an audit.

    We need to have a system to recall any patient with diabetes whose peripheral foot pulses have not been recorded in the last ten months (and do not have an appointment in the next two months) to the diabetic clinic.

- *Agree how to make changes*: the team decides who will do what, when, where, how.

  The reception/appointment staff will make an appointment and recall any patient with diabetes whose peripheral foot pulses have not been recorded in the last ten months (and do not have an appointment in the next two months) to the diabetic clinic.
  The Electronic Patient Record (EPR) will be set up to remind the diabetic nurses to assess the patient's feet at an annual appointment.

- *Reassess*: re-audit at a set interval. If things are consistent after a few six monthly or annual audits, then the interval between reassessments may be lengthened. However, don't let your standard become a fixed target, increase your standards.

  We will repeat the audit in six months to see if the changes we have made result in us being on line to meet our standard. Once we meet 90% we will change our standard to achieve 95%.

Clinical governance

When the New Labour government came into office in 1997, it expanded the parameters from audit to Clinical Governance:

Clinical governance is a system through which NHS organisations are accountable for continuously improving the quality of their services and safeguarding high standards of care by creating an environment in which excellence in clinical care will flourish.

(DH, 1998, p33)

Audit alone hadn't brought about the improvement in the provision of healthcare that the government wanted. In 2001 the DH, through the National Patient Safety Agency document *Doing Less Harm,* identified:

- 850,000 serious adverse healthcare events occurred in NHS hospitals every year;
- these cost over £2bn;
- half of these events were preventable.

Governance is the process by which an organisation publicly demonstrates that it is doing all that is reasonably practicable to manage the risks it faces. Corporate Governance applies to how public sector organisations provide transparency in their workings, including managing their funding. *Clinical* Governance was introduced to provide transparency in our *clinical* work and procedures.

Many hospitals have Clinical Governance Departments and/or Teams. In many circumstances these teams have integrated risk management team functions within them. Risk is generally defined as the probability of incurring misfortune or loss and is associated with people, buildings, estate, property, equipment, consumables, systems and management.

Risk management is a proactive approach, which aims to identify, assess and prioritise all risks, with the aim of minimising negative consequences. It is an integral function of corporate, organisational, clinical and financial governance. The risk assessment process has six identifiable stages and three extra aspects of cost benefit analysis.

Risk management

1 Identify known or potential hazards.

2 Analyse the risks.

3 Prioritise.

4 Control measures to minimise risk.

5 Implement.

6   Monitor and review.

Cost benefit analysis

1 Must be taken into account for all control measures.

2 Must be weighed against potential for adverse outcomes.

3 Risk management is a good financial investment.

Clinical governance encompasses both quality improvement *and* accountability and should be regarded as a local system of self-regulation, which underpins a national framework of revalidation for individual doctors. It is a vehicle for continuously improving the quality of patient care *and* for developing the capacity of the NHS to maintain high standards – including dealing with poor professional performance.

Clinical governance requires an organisation-wide transformation in which clinical leadership and positive organisational cultures are particularly important. Communication across the NHS is needed which involves sharing success stories as well as learning from mistakes. It must be integrated into all aspects of the delivery and provision of care and not be an optional 'add-on' which is done by the clinical governance team. It should be part of the everyday activity of all staff to ensure we have a workforce which can deliver high-quality care. It requires us to take the long view, and not allow short-term objectives to cloud the picture.

Case study 5.2: Clinical governance is part of everyday practice

A student noticed that staff seeing patients in four bedded wards were complying with most infection control policies; for example, not wearing neck ties, not sitting on beds, washing hands between patients, etc. However, staff were not routinely cleaning their stethoscopes between patients. Ten stethoscopes were selected at random for swabbing. The swabs were cultured for growth in the laboratory and it was found that all ten carried *staph. Aureus*. Sterilising materials and equipment for cleaning stethoscopes was kept at the nursing station. There is a sink in each four bedded ward that all the staff use to wash their hands. The student suggested putting stethoscope cleaning equipment by the sink in each four bedded ward. Subsequent observation showed staff using the cleaning equipment on their stethoscopes and cultures from a repeat random swabbing show no organism growth.

Critical Incidence Reporting is a key function within Clinical Governance as it is essential that we learn from events that should not have happened to patients, including those that nearly go wrong. When serious incidents occur which lead to permanent harm or death related to the incident, then an incident investigation must be carried out. These are often referred to as Serious Untoward Incident (SUI) investigations. The Intensive Care Society explains a critical incident as:

> any event or circumstance that caused or could have caused (referred to as a near miss) unplanned harm, suffering, loss or damage. Examples include: an event or omission that has arisen during clinical care and has caused physical or psychological injury to a patient, drug errors (failure of proper identification, inaccurate dosage etc.) which cause actual or potential harm to the patient, or incidents of slips, trips or falls.
>
> **(www.ics.ac.uk/intensive_care_professional/standards_and_**
> **guidelines/critical_incident_reporting_2006)**

There are a number of documents which can guide you through Critical Incident Reporting from the *NHS Evidence – National Library of Guidelines* (**www.library. nhs.uk**). In addition Root Cause Analysis (RCA) is one of the nationally recognised approaches to incident investigation throughout the NHS. It is a logical tool to investigate the 'what, how and why' of an incident. The National Patient Safety Agency (NPSA) has produced a tool kit (available at **www.msnpsa.nhs.uk/rcatoolkit/ course/iindex.htm**) which takes you through the methodology.

ACTIVITY 5.2 THE NPSA TOOLKIT AND ADVERSE INCIDENTS

Go to **www.scps.org.uk/pdfs/GrittenReport.pdf** and read the 2005 Gritten Report into *The Adverse incident that lead to the death of a paediatric cardiac surgery patient at United Bristol Healthcare NHS Trust on 27 May 2005.*

Reflect on how the NPSA tool kit was used for this large-scale incident.

Best practice

All health professionals are challenged to undertake 'best practice', but this phrase is often used unrelated to any evidence base. It implies that you personally need to know everything to be able to carry out best practice instinctively based on your knowledge and experience. This is complicated by professional arguments about clinical independence – being allowed to take the best clinical decision for the patient. Clear evidence exists on what is best practice for many clinical conditions, and hopefully, protocols are based on the evidence.

There are many ways of breaking down aspects of care for measuring whether we are providing a quality service. Department of Health documents regularly present the facets of care that they want improving, using the six components of quality identified by Robert J. Maxwell, when he was Director of The King's Fund:

1 Access
2 Relevance to need
3 Effectiveness
4 Equity
5 Acceptability
6 Efficiency

(Maxwell, 1984)

I consider these components a good guide for breaking the care we provide into relevant elements; however, I have always felt there should be a seventh component of quality:

7 Humanity

If you undertake one to six without humanity you won't be providing good care.

However, this doesn't tell us how to actually provide best practice. Nor does this define what quality is. There is only one word for quality and each of us can interpret it slightly differently. If you think of shopping for baked beans – how do you know that you have bought quality? It could be a number of things:

- cost;

- brand;

- sugar content;

- bean to sauce ratio;

- type/quantity of spice and herb extracts;

- taste.

People often argue that products need to 'meet expectations' but beware of this as a measure of quality. If you expect the beans to be tasteless and they are, then you have not bought quality beans, though your expectations have been met. What it actually comes down to is 'do you like them?' Can you eat them? If you don't like them, you won't eat them – so they won't be fit for purpose – which means, for you, they aren't quality.

We can apply the simple measure of 'fit for purpose' to measure quality in healthcare. Did you safely and humanely fulfil the requirements and needs of your patients? If so, you are fit for purpose. What best practice and clinical protocols aim to do is provide evidence-based tools to enable you to provide care that is at least fit for purpose. Being an independent clinical practitioner gives you the space to do more than be just fit for purpose, to enable you to provide more than best practice when it is necessary for a specific patient.

ACTIVITY 5.3 EVIDENCE-BASED PRACTICE

Go to **www.patientvoices.org.uk/flv/0119pv384.htm** and watch the film *Nil by Mouth*.

How do you find the most up-to-date, evidence-based information to make sure you give patients accurate information and to prevent confusion?

To undertake best practice it has become obvious that we have reached a point in many parts of our lives, when what we do is too complicated to just remember. As Atul Gawande argues:

> We have accumulated stupendous know-how. . . . Nonetheless, that know-how is often unmanageable. Avoidable failures are common and persistent. . . . And the reason is increasingly evident: the volume and complexity of what we know has exceeded our individual ability to deliver its benefits correctly, safely, or reliably.
>
> (Gawande, 2010, p13)

This applies to what could be considered basic, routine procedures. Gawande (2010) gives the example of monitoring whether well-trained doctors undertook five basic steps to prevent infections when inserting a central line:

1 Hand washing.

2 Cleaning patient's skin with chlorhexidine.

3 Covering the entire patient with sterile drapes.

4 Wearing a mask, hat, sterile gown and gloves.

5 Once the line is in, covering the insertion site with a sterile dressing.

When observed, it was found that doctors missed at least one step in a third of patients. This resulted in the check list being introduced to actually be 'checked' – that is, the doctors were no longer only observed, they were reminded if they didn't follow all five actions. Within a year the infection rate dropped from 11 percent to 0 – preventing 43 infections, eight deaths and saving $2 million.

There is no need for us to over-complicate our lives and try to remember every step. Consider airline pilots whose routines are often not as complex as ours yet who have regular check lists designed to improve safety. Berwick and Leape (1999) compared the figures for aerospace versus North American healthcare. Between 1990 and 1994, USA airline fatalities were 0.27 per 1,000,000 aircraft departures. While studies of healthcare in the USA at the same time showed that in two highly regarded hospitals, serious or potentially serious medication errors occur for 6.7 per cent of patients and the Harvard Medical Practice Study (review of over 30,000 hospital records in New York state) found adverse events occur in 3.7 per cent of hospital admissions, over half were preventable and 13.6 per cent of which died. UK statistics are comparable (Berwick and Leape, 1999).

The World Health Organisation (WHO) has introduced the 'Surgical Safety Checklist' with the aim that it will be adopted in operating theatres worldwide in order to reduce medical errors. Wherever the checklist has been introduced, it has prevented mistakes, whether it is 'Has antibiotic prophylaxis been given within the last 60 minutes?' or 'That instrument, sponge and needle counts are correct' (World Alliance for Patient Safety, 2008)

ACTIVITY 5.4 THE SURGICAL SAFETY CHECKLIST

Go to **www.who.int/patientsafety/safesurgery/ss_checklist/en/index.html** and read the 'WHO surgical safety checklist' and ideally the 'Implementation Manual'.

Investigate whether it is used in your local hospital operating theatres. If not, ask the theatre manager why not.

Service improvement

The fundamental of service improvement is focusing on the processes and not blaming others. To paraphrase Berwick: 'Every system is perfectly designed to produce the outcome it achieves' (1999). It is essential we know the system is right because until we get the processes working properly, we cannot know whether or not people are doing things properly. There are four basic steps for understanding our processes as shown in Figure 5.3.

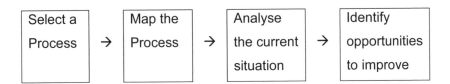

Figure 5.3 Four basic steps for understanding our processes

Mapping the process can be a simple flow chart of what is actually happening and no more complicated than a recipe for a cake: what are the ingredients needed (the staff and the equipment) and what do you do with them? Once you have all the steps you can see where there is repetition, delays or bottlenecks. To improve the situation you need to make sure your process has as few steps as possible, each step must be useful and add value to the process. Most mistakes happen at a 'hand over': the extra step in a process. We also tend to over-complicate our procedures. When something new is introduced we add it to an already complex situation instead of investigating whether it can replace an existing stage. The simpler the process and fewer steps, the less chance there is to make mistakes.

However, one of the biggest problems people find is identifying the actual process to map because our systems are so complex. People tend to set grand aims, such as 'to improve the quality of care to people undergoing total hip replacements so that they receive the care they need'.

This is a wonderful ambition – but what needs improving? It is necessary to hone down on specific issues that don't work as well as they should, such as 'Providing appropriate information to patients and carers when they need it' or 'streamlining the pre-admission assessment' or 'making sure the patient gets pre-surgery antibiotics' or 'improving the delivery of drugs from pharmacy to prevent discharge delays'.

A *Model for Improvement* (see Figure 5.4) developed by Langley et al. (1996, cited in NHS Institute 2007) is helpful in focusing on what you want to do. By answering the three fundamental questions for improvement we can be specific about what it is we are attempting to do. Measurement is essential because while all improvement requires change, not all change is an improvement. However, measurement does not always require statistical analysis, it can be as basic as 'what will we see that is different?' Seeking and using the ideas and hunches from the staff team involved in the issues is normally the easiest way of finding solutions to the 'problems'.

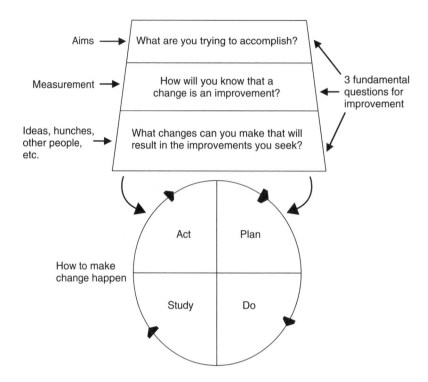

Figure 5.4 A model for improvement

Source: Langley et al. 1996, cited in NHS Institute, 2007, p31

The plan–do–study–act (PDSA) cycle was developed by Edward Deming in the early 1900s and is a basic, validated, successful tool for change.

Plan   the objective, the plan to carry out the cycle (who, what, where, when) and the plan for studying what impact the change has.

Do   'just do it' – carry out the plan, document any problems or unexpected observations and begin analysis of the 'data'.

Study   complete the analysis of the 'data' to see whether the change created the outcome you were aiming for and summarise what was learned.

Act   decide what changes need to be made – if the change was successful, embed it into everyday reality – if it did not quite do what you wanted, plan another change and start the next cycle.

If you compare the processes of the audit cycle with the model for improvement, you can see how they logically fit together, by bringing the basic data together with a method for making the changes. Monitoring and improving care is the responsibility of all healthcare professionals and using tools that assist the process helps to make this more systematic.

Case study 5.3: A team approach to improving hydration for stroke patients

In a Stroke Unit, it had been noted that there was a high use of saline drips to prevent dehydration. The initial response from the staff was that this was raised as a cost-cutting measure; however, it was pointed out that the incidence of infection following the insertion of a drips was high. The team initially thought they should improve care by trying to reduce infections following the insertion of a saline drip; however, one of the physiotherapists in the team pointed out that the drips also reduced their ability to improve patients' mobility.

Following discussion, the team agreed that what they were trying to achieve was 'a reduction in the use of saline drips to manage the lack of fluid intake, while maintaining the appropriate level of hydration in their patients'. They would know if a change was an improvement because they would be administering fewer drips and patients would not be dehydrated.

A nurse suggested providing patients with their favourite soft drink, instead of just offering water or weak orange squash.

The first PDSA cycle was to ask patients what their favourite soft drink was. If the patient was unable to speak, a close relative was asked. When this was studied, it was found that the hospital order-ing system was too slow to get the various soft drinks (e.g. apple juice and soda water) in place in time to maintain appropriate levels of hydration.

Another member of the team suggested asking visitors to provide the drinks until they could get them ordered. This was done and they instantly noticed the number of patients taking fluids voluntarily went up and the number of drips inserted was reduced.

Over a six month period the team had reduced the use of saline drips by 73 per cent while maintaining appropriate hydration levels. They also had a consequential reduction in infections and the need to administer antibiotics. The financial savings were so great that they were able to buy a fridge and keep it stocked with a range of the most popularly requested soft drinks.

Chapter summary

This chapter has:

- described the policy drivers behind monitoring care and improving service;

- reminded you to focus on the patient and understand care from the service user perspective;

- outlined the audit cycle and how to set standards against which improvement can be monitored;

- described clinical governance and the role of risk management, root cause analysis and critical incidence reporting;

- discussed Best Practice to provide quality care and the role of protocols, checklists and guidelines;

- contextualised service improvement as part of an overriding approach to the provision of care and the importance of focusing on the processes.

GOING FURTHER

Gawande, A (2010) *The Checklist Manifesto: How to Get Things Right.* London: Profile Books.
   This is an enjoyable, easy read that clearly explains the benefits of using simple checklists to improve care and prevent mistakes.

NHS Institute (2007) *The Improvement Leaders' Guides.* The NHS Institute for Innovation and Improvement. Available on line at **www.institute.nhs. uk/improvementleadersguide**
   Further information can be found in detail within the *Improvement Leaders' Guides.* These are very useful small guides that have been brought together to aid all healthcare professionals with the issues relating to improvement. They are split into three sections covering *General Improvement Skills, Process and Systems Thinking* and *Personal and Organisational Development.* They are currently available free to all NHS employees and online at above address.

Scholtes, PR, Joiner, BL and Streibel, JL (2003) *The Team Handbook,* 3rd edition. Madison, WI: Oriel Inc.
   The Team Handbook includes much that is relevant to anyone wanting to lead change and serve our customer (patients/service users/carers) better. It helps you to apply tools and concepts by using worksheets and templates throughout the book.

chapter 6

Patient Safety

Nicola Cooper and Alison Cracknell

Achieving foundation competences

This chapter will help you to begin to meet the following requirements of the *Foundation Programme Curriculum* (2010).

Outcome 7 Patient safety within clinical governance

Demonstrates a clear commitment to maintaining patient safety and delivering high-quality reliable care.

- Makes patient safety a priority in own clinical practice:

  - identifies and minimises potential risks and main hazards to patients;
  - delivers protocol-driven care;
  - describes a critical incident and methods of preventing an adverse event.

- Promotes patient safety through good team-working:

  - cross-checks instructions and actions with colleagues, for example, medicines to be injected;
  - draws attention to risks or potential risks to patients regardless of status of colleagues;
  - describes ways of identifying and dealing with poor performance in self and colleagues, including senior colleagues.

Understands the principles of quality and safety improvement:

  - demonstrates knowledge of how and when to report adverse events and 'near misses' to local and, where appropriate, national reporting systems;
  - describes opportunities for improving the reliability of care following adverse events or 'near misses';
  - describes root-cause analysis.

Knowledge

- The nature of human error and the importance of systems factors in relation to patient safety.
- Principles of the investigation and analysis of adverse events and patient safety incidents as a means to making care safer.

Chapter overview

Modern healthcare is complex. When things go wrong, it is not necessarily because an incompetent healthcare professional 'made a mistake', rather it is because the successful treatment of each patient depends on a wide range of factors that is the healthcare system itself.

In recent years, we have come to understand that healthcare systems in developed countries cause harm to patients. Research over the last 20 years has consistently shown that 10 per cent of hospital in-patients are harmed by Western health-care systems, and in 1 per cent of these cases this directly leads to their death (Brennan et al., 1991; Wilson et al., 1995; Vincent et al., 2001; Sari et al., 2007). This equates to over 100,000 deaths a year in the UK. Just imagine if you or one of your relatives were admitted to hospital and told that you had a one in a 100 chance of dying from something not related to your reason for admission, but because of an error.

Sometimes this harm could not have been prevented – for example, an allergic reaction to a drug in a patient with no known allergies. But at least half of all harm is preventable, whether this is through medication errors, failure to act on seriously abnormal vital signs, hospital associated infections, or failure to prescribe treatments to prevent deep vein thrombosis.

After reading this chapter you will be able to:

- recognise that modern healthcare is a 'high risk' industry;
- identify the principal threats to patient safety and how you can act to minimise them;
- effectively communicate with colleagues to ensure patient safety;
- participate in incident reporting and learning from errors.

Errors in healthcare

'Error' is a technical term in industry meaning an unintended event that could have caused harm. In healthcare, we term this a 'patient safety incident'. Serious incidents are just the tip of the iceberg. There are far more minor incidents and 'near misses' that show just how unsafe the systems we work in can be (see Figure 6.1).

In industry, it has been estimated that for every major injury there are 29 minor injuries and 300 'no harm' accidents (Heinreich et al., 1980). Although incidents are less likely to get reported when a patient has not come to any harm, incident reporting is important because we can learn far more about how to improve our systems from the greater number of 'no harm' accidents than we can from the smaller number of serious incidents that occur.

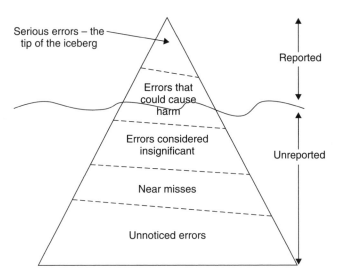

Figure 6.1 The adverse incident 'iceberg'

Source: Cooper et al., 2006

In one year, serious incidents cost the NHS £2 billion in additional hospital stay alone (DH, 2000), and even more in negligence claims. Safer care is not only better quality care, it costs less.

Other 'high-risk' industries, such as commercial aviation and the oil and gas industries, have studied error and serious incidents and have developed systems and training to reduce incidents to a minimum. Healthcare is catching up when it comes to learning about error and implementing systems and training to minimise harm to patients.

Box 6.1 Definitions

- An *adverse event* is an unintended injury caused by the healthcare system. An adverse event can occur because of things we do or things we do not do, and may or may not be preventable.
- A *patient safety incident* (or error) refers to an unintended event caused by the healthcare system which may or may not have led to harm, and includes near misses.

How things go wrong

Errors are inevitable in a highly complex system such as modern healthcare. The majority of healthcare staff do not come to work to deliberately harm patients – rather 'to err is human'. Even if a 600-bed hospital managed to eliminate medication errors by 99.9 per cent there would still be 4,000 medication errors each year

(Leape, 1994). However, research shows that errors are predictable and tend to repeat themselves in patterns. The system in which we work can either adapt for this and make patient safety incidents less likely, or it can in fact create 'accidents waiting to happen'.

If healthcare professionals understand that errors are predictable most of the time, then they can adapt their behaviour to minimise them.

James Reason (2000) summarises the research in to *how* things go wrong with the 'Swiss cheese' model of accident causation. Let us use the example of blood transfusion. Every organisation has successive layers of defences, barriers and safe-guards – from donation to testing, treatment, storage and eventually administration on a ward. However, because humans are involved, these defences can have 'holes' in them. Some of these holes are organisational – for example, if the hospital does not have a standard operating procedure for blood transfusion and does not require all staff to be trained before administering blood products. These are 'latent holes'. Other holes are 'active holes', usually at the point of care – for example, staff may deliberately take a short cut or make a mistake, such as mislabelling the blood cross match. On any particular day, all these holes can align and lead to a serious patient safety incident, such as a transfusion reaction or death.

Examples of latent holes include insufficient staffing, inadequate training, low standards of quality and inadequate technology. Examples of active holes include slips and distractions, lapses, mistakes or failure in judgement often due to insufficient knowledge and violations of protocols.

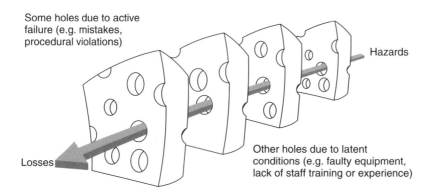

Figure 6.2 The 'Swiss cheese' model of accident causation. © James Reason

---

ACTIVITY 6.1 IDENTIFYING THE HOLES

Look at the Swiss cheese model above. Can you think of an adverse event which you know about and what the latent and active holes were in that situation?

Box 6.2 *Key concepts in patient safety*

- Errors are inevitable in a complex system such as healthcare.
- Errors within the healthcare system are predictable and tend to repeat them-selves in patterns.
- We should all expect and anticipate errors.
- Reporting clinical incidents and near misses is the main way in which an organisa-tion can learn and change.
- Everyone has a part to play in making our systems safer.

Human factors

'Human factors' describes the study of how we can adapt our behaviour to minimise patient safety incidents. All pilots have to pass a human factors exam. But doctors and other healthcare professionals, who work in equally high-risk occupations, might never even have heard of this term.

The study of human factors includes:

- understanding the scale and nature of error in healthcare;

- situation awareness;

- the limitations of human performance;

- communication in teams.

Pilots also adhere to an anonymous compulsory incident reporting system, and are required to adhere to strict communication protocols. They also regularly use checklists – an important means of ensuring safety.

Situation awareness

Situation awareness refers to knowing what is going on around you and being alert to potential problems. An individual can have situation awareness, but it is important that the whole team is also aware. For example, you may be in a peri-arrest situation, and a team member is obtaining an arterial blood gas, but you notice the patient has an airway obstruction. It is important to state the obvious, *because what seems obvious to you is not necessarily obvious to everyone else*. Often, a team's situation awareness can be low because nobody communicates.

Situation awareness is compromised by:

- poor/conflicting information or communication;

- confusion (e.g. over roles and responsibilities);

- departure from standard procedures;
- distractions;
- inexperience;
- poor training;
- poor interpersonal skills or attitude;
- physical and emotional fatigue and stress.

It is now common practice in theatres in the UK to have a 'time out' before starting an operation as well as a team brief before the theatre list start. This is so that all team members are ready to anticipate problems and are aware of what kit will be required. Each member of the team has to confirm that they agree it is the correct patient, the correct procedure and the correct site before surgery starts. If the patient is having local anaesthesia, he or she has to agree as well! This practice was introduced because analysis of cases of 'wrong site surgery' showed that in nearly every case, there was someone in theatre who knew it was the wrong site, but did not feel able to speak up. Never be afraid to state the obvious.

Case study 6.1: Removal of the wrong kidney and failure to speak out

Mr Z, a 70-year-old man, died shortly after surgeons removed the one healthy kidney rather than the diseased kidney during an operation at Prince Philip Hospital, Llanelli in 2000.

- How could this have happened?

The X-rays of Mr Z were displayed the wrong way round in theatre.

- How this could have happened?
- How could it have been prevented?

One person in the theatre knew that the surgeon was removing the wrong kidney.
- Why did the error still occur?

It was the medical student in theatre who knew the wrong kidney was being removed.

- Does this change the need to communicate the potential for error?
- Why didn't anything get said or why wasn't it heard?

The limitations of human performance

Many doctors strive to be perfect. It is vital to understand that perfection is impossible. 'To err is human' – this is basic psychology, and proven again and again in experiments. Studies of doctors working night shifts show their performance deteriorates after nearly 24 hours without sleep to the equivalent of being 'over the limit' in terms of blood alcohol levels.

Human performance is affected by workload, distractions, stress, hunger, fatigue and illness among other things. A common example of how humans predictably err is the cash point machine, or ATM. Some ATMs give you your cash before returning your card. A significant percentage of people forget their card after they have taken their cash, and rely on the honesty of the person behind them in the queue to let them know of their error. Newer ATMs have employed a concept called 'human factors engineering' and return your card first. A message is displayed: 'Please take your card before receiving your cash'. This ensures that the predictable human behaviour of leaving their card behind is reduced.

Human factors engineering involves designing systems that account for the predictability of fallible human nature. We are forgetful, tired, distracted, busy and sometimes have a bad day. Healthcare professionals need to understand this and act with this in mind. Good healthcare *processes* are deliberately designed with human factors in mind. Standard operating procedures and checklists are examples of ways in which healthcare processes can be made safer.

On an individual level, James Reason proposed a '3-bucket' model to help healthcare staff understand their own limitations before starting a new task (Figure 6.3). There are three factors to consider: yourself, the context and the task. If I ask you to insert a cannula in a compliant patient with large veins at the start of a day shift, you are unlikely to anticipate any problems. But suppose the patient is Hepatitis C positive, uncooperative, an intravenous drug user with poor veins, it is the middle of the night and you are hungry – you can anticipate that your buckets are 'full'. In this case, you should stop and consider the situation before deciding how best to proceed.

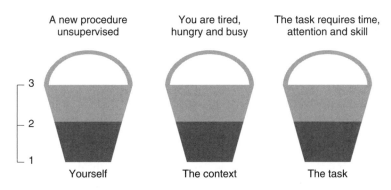

Figure 6.3 Reason's '3 bucket' model. © James Reason, 2006

Good healthcare professionals are not those who do not make mistakes. Good healthcare professionals are those who expect to make mistakes and act on that expectation.

(Reason, 2006)

How can we adapt for the limitations of human performance? It is a fact that healthcare staff routinely break rules and ignore reasonable procedures designed to ensure patient safety. One way of ensuring patient safety is by *observing rules and conscientiously following standard operating procedures.* We all have to take personal responsibility for our actions.

In one survey, 75 per cent of pilots said that fatigue affected their performance but only 30 per cent of surgeons said the same (McAllister, 1997). If we are aware of the fact that there are limitations to human performance, we can act safely. Sometimes in healthcare, we are guilty of 'dangerous benevolence'. This means that we are always trying to help our patients, so we often cut corners in order to do so, without first thinking through the patient safety implications.

Communication in teams

Effective communication in teams is a basic pre-requisite of patient safety. A recent study on an Acute Medical Unit showed how interruptions were commonplace, and how junior doctors frequently failed to indicate that they could not hear or understand an instruction properly. Ambiguous pronouns were commonly used – for example, 'he', 'she', 'it', 'they', 'the man in bed 1' (Hassan et al., 2009).

Poor communication is found to be a key factor in the majority of serious incidents when they are analysed after the event. Effective communication includes:

- confirming roles and responsibilities;
- communicating plans;
- stating the obvious;
- avoiding ambiguous terms such as 'he', 'she', 'it', 'they';
- giving clear instructions;
- using 'readback' (the practice of repeating back to ensure you heard correctly);
- verbalising concerns;
- calling for help if needed;
- listening to others;
- co-operating.

For example, one of the authors works in an Acute Medical Unit where the doctors take it in turns to work shifts on the unit, so they may be unfamiliar with how things work. There is a mandatory 8 a.m. team brief before the ward round starts, during which everyone has to introduce their name and grade, then the way the unit works is explained to them.

Other simple communication protocols include SBARR – recommended by the Patient Safety First Campaign (UK). SBARR stands for Situation, Background, Assessment, Recommendation and then Readback. This is particularly recommended when communicating information about sick patients, but is useful for any situation, including the post-take ward round. Using SBARR has been shown to improve the effectiveness of communication and takes less time. Many junior doctors call their seniors with a situation and a background, but fail to accurately communicate what they think is going on and what they really want their senior to do next. Using SBARR helps to structure the conversation so nothing is missed.

Box 6.3 SBARR

- Situation

  - *What is happening now*
  - 'I am on ward 39 with a sick patient and need assistance.'

- Background

  - *Circumstances leading up to this*
  - 'He's 40 years old, admitted with a diabetic foot ulcer, now his MEWS is 6, he is normally fit and well.'

- Assessment

  - *What you think the problem is*
  - 'He appears to have severe sepsis.'

- Recommendation

  - *What you would like to happen next*
  - 'I've started the severe sepsis resuscitation care bundle, but he needs a senior doctor to see him as soon as possible.'

Red flags

It was obvious to everyone that things were going seriously wrong, but no-one liked to mention it!

(From an air accident investigation)

A 'red flag' is a term we use to mean a 'warning'. These often occur in the minutes leading up to a serious patient safety incident. Examples of red flags include:

- confusion;

- conflicting information;

- lack of information;

- departure from standard procedure;

- unease;

- denial or irritability;

- inaction;

- alarms going off;

- alarming thoughts.

A red flag is a *cue for action*. It means you have to stop to communicate with the rest of the team so that the situation can be re-assessed and a decision can be made on how to proceed.

Look at the list above. Have you ever experienced a 'red flag' moment?

For example, if a patient is taken to theatre, but the notes are missing, that lack of information is a red flag or warning that something is likely to go wrong. Or imagine a porter is taking a patient for a procedure and he says, 'Just mind your arms Ethel,' but the patient replies, 'Actually my name is Edna.' That is also a red flag. Or imagine you have a very sick patient on the ward but your bleep to a senior colleague is not being answered. That is another red flag.

The 'PACE' system of graded assertiveness of how to communicate is useful when you come across a red flag:

P = probing

A = alerting

C = challenging

E = emergency stop.

It is a way of communicating to the rest of the team, starting gently and becoming more assertive if necessary.

PACE – graded assertiveness:

- *Probe* – 'Do you know that . . .?'

- *Alert* – 'Can we re-assess the situation . . .?'

- *Challenge* – 'Please stop what you are doing for a minute while . . .'

- *Emergency!* – 'Wait, STOP what you are doing!'

Pilots are almost unanimous in saying that junior members of a team should always question decisions made by senior members where safety is concerned. Unfortunately, the effect of hierarchy in healthcare means that we do not always have the same attitude, but this is changing.

Reporting and learning from errors

Referring back to the 'Swiss cheese' model of accident causation, imagine you lived in a log cabin next to a swamp full of mosquitoes. You will never stop being bitten by swatting individual mosquitoes every day. You need to drain the swamp. In the same way, when it comes to errors and serious incidents, we need to look at the 'root causes' in order to stop the same thing from happening again and again. You may have heard of the term 'root cause analysis'. This is when an adverse event is investigated by looking at the holes further back in the system which are often as (or more) important in terms of prevention than the obvious errors that occurred at the point of care.

An organisation that prepares for inevitable errors and knows how to deal with them when they do occur is also safer. A simple example is that every area which uses morphine and midazolam injections should also stock the drugs for reversing their effects, such as naloxone and flumazenil. As a doctor, you should always anticipate what could go wrong and be prepared for it.

Reporting near misses and patient safety incidents is the main way that an organisation can learn how its systems can be changed for the better to prevent future harm. There are two main incident reporting systems in the National Health Service. One is the routine incident reporting system that is generally ward or unit based. The other is for 'serious untoward incidents' that require a different form to be completed and are usually investigated by trained incident investigators within the hospital. A serious untoward incident would be death or major harm caused, for example, by an error. As a junior doctor, you should approach your line manager (consultant) or clinical director to flag up a potential serious untoward incident in the first instance.

Here are some examples of the sort of routine incidents that should be reported:

- medication errors (including intravenous fluids);
- adverse drug reactions (which should also be reported online or using the Yellow Card system in the back of the BNF);
- equipment faults or equipment not available;
- patient injury as a result of a procedure (which may be a recognised complication);
- care not as intended;
- patient care adversely affected for non-clinical reasons (e.g. ICU patients who are transferred due to lack of beds);
- injuries (including falls and needle stick);
- assault.

Case study 6.2: The end of a shift

Chloe was nearing the end of her shift and was tired and hungry. She was asked to write up the evening warfarin doses, which she did before she rushed off as she was already late for her lift home.

The next day she was asked by the pharmacist why she had written up 10 mg of warfarin for Mr Patel when he had an INR of 4.5?

Chloe was mortified; she had not checked the blood results from that day before prescribing the warfarin.

What to do if you are involved in an adverse incident

There are a series of generic steps to follow if you are involved in an incident.

- Report the incident to your senior immediately, ensure safety of the patient and any immediate management that is necessary is commenced.

- Arrange for your senior to inform patient/carer of the event.

- Complete an incident form.

- Consider the impact on the rest of shift. If it was catastrophic, for example a death in theatre, staff involved should have a time out and not just carry on with the list.

- Comply with filling out any statement and reports that may be required for organisational investigation.

- Recognise the potential impact on yourself, other staff, patient and carers.

- Reflect in your e-portfolio, how the incident has changed your practice and that of the team or unit.

So recall Case study 6.2: The end of a shift. What clinical steps will Chloe have to do? How could this be avoided in the future? Some wards already have 'barriers' in place to stop this happening. What are they in your place of work?

ACTIVITY 6.2 INCIDENT REPORTING

- When was the last time you filled in an incident form?
- When was the last time you could have filled in an incident form?
- Why did you not fill in a form?

In the past, before we really understood about the nature of error, healthcare organisations tended simply to blame people when things went wrong. This approach is like swatting individual mosquitoes around a swamp, as described earlier. Healthcare is moving towards a new approach – a fair, reporting and learning culture which recognises how errors occur and how they can be prevented. Personal responsibility is still important when it comes to patient safety. But research shows that to prevent the same thing from happening again, we usually need to look further.

The way we have traditionally managed failures and mistakes in healthcare has been called the person approach – we single out the individuals involved at the time of the incident and hold them accountable. Our tendency to 'blame' is thought to be one of the main constraints on the health system's ability to manage risk and improve as a result of error.

Other high-risk industries now realise that a blame culture will not bring safety issues to the surface. Organisations that place a premium on safety routinely examine all aspects of the system in the event of an accident, including equipment design, procedures, training and organisational features. Using a systems approach to error does not imply a 'blame free' culture. The entire system of care is examined to find out what went wrong rather than focusing on who did it. Only after careful attention to the multiple factors associated with the incident can there be an assessment as to whether individuals need to be held accountable. Individual healthcare professionals *are* required to be accountable for their actions, maintain competence and practise ethically.

Making small improvements

As a junior doctor, you are ideally placed to see the potential for 'accidents waiting to happen' in your workplace and may have some ideas as to how things could be changed to improve matters.

Start by talking your idea through with colleagues, then go and speak to the ward/unit manager or clinical director with your concerns and proposal. Small improvements can be made using the plan–do–study–act cycle. In other words, come up with an idea, try it out, see if it works, and then go for it if it does or change it if it does not (see Chapter 5 for more on the cycle).

Experience in successful organisations shows that when everyone is empowered to suggest small changes that make a difference, that organisation is likely to be safer – as well as a more satisfying place to work.

Box 6.4 Five myths about patient safety

Here are five myths about human error and its management:

- Errors are random and highly variable.
- Bad errors are made by bad people.
- Practice makes perfect.
- Errors by highly trained professionals are rare.
- It is easier to change people than systems.

What's the evidence?

There is a lot of evidence that specific interventions to reduce harm, such as those aimed at preventing falls or monitoring and treating the deteriorating adult, do work. However, much time and effort is given over to large-scale national systematic initiatives – do these interventions make a difference in patient care and outcomes?

A research article published in the *British Medical Journal* specifically looked at answering this question. The study emphasises that quality improvement interventions tackling specific issues such as hospital acquired infection are easier to demonstrate change than that of systemic change in large organisations. There were generic safety improvements irrespective of the specific intervention.

They concluded:

- Patient safety has improved across the NHS on many of the measures used in our study of English hospitals;
- No additional effect of the Safer Patients Initiative could be detected;
- Several possible explanations for the absence of an additional effect of the programme can be offered, including a 'rising tide' phenomenon where improvements in patient safety were driven by common forces across the NHS.

(Benning et al., 2011, p342)

Chapter summary

Individual doctors and nurses can improve patient safety by engaging with patients and their families, checking procedures, learning from errors and communicating effectively with the whole healthcare team. Such activities can also save costs because they minimise the harm caused to patients. When errors are reported and analysed they can help identify the main contributing factors. Understanding the factors that lead to errors is essential for developing changes that will prevent errors from being made.

GOING FURTHER

Department of Health (2000) *An Organisation with a Memory. Report of an Expert Group on Learning from Adverse Events in the NHS.* London: DH. www.dh.gov.uk

Vincent, Charles (2005) *Patient Safety.* London: Churchill Livingstone.
    A really good introductory text.

National Patient Safety Agency **www.npsa.nhs.uk**
> Provides useful improvement resources and includes the National Reporting and Learning Service.

WHO Patient Safety Curriculum Guide for Medical Schools **www.who.int/patient-safety/activities/technical/medical_curriculum/en/index.html**
> Resource for delivery of patient safety education to medical students and junior doctors.

Patient Safety First Campaign **www.patientsafetyfirst.nhs.uk/content.aspx?path=/**
> Has the aim of changing the culture within the NHS to ensure that it makes patient safety its first priority with no avoidable death.

The Institute for Healthcare Improvement **www.ihi.org/ihi**
> Resources on many dimensions of healthcare improvement and patient safety.

Sanders, J and Cook, G (2007) *ABC of Patient Safety*. London: BMJ Books/Blackwell Publishing.

chapter 7

Relationship Building with Patients and Carers

John Spencer

Achieving foundation competences

This chapter will help you to begin to meet the following requirements of the *Foundation Programme Curriculum* (2010).

2. Good clinical care
Eliciting a history
Outcome: demonstrates the knowledge, attitudes, behaviours, skills and competences to be able to take a history

Competences

- Takes accomplished, concise, targeted history and communicate in complex situations which include:

  - clinical;
  - psychological;
  - social and personal;
  - the patient's personal factors.

- Takes account of background where relevant and appropriate, including verbal and non-verbal cues.
- Takes a focused family history, and constructs and interprets a family tree where relevant.
- Obtains collateral history when available.
- Manages three-way consultations.

6. Relationship with patients and communication skills
Within a consultation
Outcome: demonstrates the knowledge, skills, attitudes and behaviours to be able to communicate effectively with patients, relatives and colleagues in the circumstances outlined below

Competences

- Is always polite and considerate to patients.
- Explains options clearly and checks understanding, encouraging patients with knowledge of their condition to make appropriately informed decisions about their care.

- Provides or recommends relevant written/online information for patients.
- Deals appropriately with angry or dissatisfied patients.

Knowledge

- How to structure the interview to identify the patient's:
  - concerns/problem list;
  - expectations;
  - understanding;
  - acceptance.

- Environments in which patients from different social and cultural backgrounds are able to talk about their health beliefs and practices, particularly when discussing different treatment options.

Chapter overview

After reading this chapter you should recognise the central importance of the patient–doctor relationship, and will be able to:

- deploy the basic micro-skills of communication more effectively;
- explore the patient's perspective with greater confidence and sense of purpose;
- explain things to patients, and involve them in decisions about their care;
- demonstrate empathy.

Context and background

> The good physician treats the disease; the great physician treats the patient who has the disease.
>
> (Sir William Osler)

To say that the doctor–patient relationship lies at the heart of clinical practice is something of an understatement. An effective relationship is the basis of the trust and empathy from which so many outcomes derive. It enables people to tell their stories, articulate their ideas, air their concerns, and vent their feelings, and potentially prevents misunderstanding and error. A recent study even found that adherence to medication depended partly upon patients' perceptions of the quality of the relationship (Stavropoulou, 2010).

The doctor–patient relationship has been described as the 'cement' that holds the consultation together, and most models of clinical communication emphasise the importance of so-called relational competence (Mouton, 2007; Silverman et al., 2005; Neighbour, 2005; Pendleton et al., 2003; Stewart et al., 2003); to quote one of the authors 'Relationships matter. It makes a difference to communication in healthcare, to the people who are involved, to healthcare and its outcomes.' (Silverman et al., 2005, p117). A relationship-centred encounter will not only be *technically* effective, but will also be informative, enable the patient to tell their story, encourage them to participate, and will respond to their feelings and concerns (Roter, 2000).

Yet survey after survey has demonstrated, in both hospital and community settings, that whilst the public puts great store by a respectful and empathic relationship and communication that is sensitive to their needs, sadly doctors often fall short in terms of meeting their expectations (Picker Institute Europe and Care Quality Commission, **www.nhssurveys.org/publications**).

It is easy to assume that attending to the doctor–patient relationship is only relevant to situations in which continuity is a key feature, such as general practice or caring for patients with long-term conditions. As it happens, it may be even *more* important in the hubbub of clinical practice in out-patients and on the wards, when contact with patients and carers is usually transitory. A brief one-off encounter between patient and doctor that goes wrong may have long lasting effects.

It may also be thought that busying oneself with relational aspects takes up valuable time at the expense of the 'real' purpose of the consultation, that is, taking a history, making a diagnosis, initiating treatment and so on. However, there is good evidence that paying deliberate attention to the relationship does not take significantly more time, and in any case it makes other consultation tasks easier to achieve.

At policy level, the General Medical Council has enshrined the importance of the patient–doctor relationship in its standards and guidelines, for both clinical practice (General Medical Council, 2006a), and education and training (General Medical Council, 2009a). The Royal College of Physicians published guidelines about communication (RCP, 1997), and highlighted the central importance of the patient–doctor relationship in its report on medical professionalism (RCP, 2005).

Recognising the fact the poor communication is a major factor in medical error and litigation, bodies such as the defence unions and the National Patient Safety Agency emphasise the centrality of communication in managing risk (see Medical Protection Society website; NPSA, 2004). These policy issues are not confined to the UK. Similar developments have been global; for example, the CANMEDS framework in Canada (CANMEDS, 2010).

This chapter explores the following areas:

- Key elements of the doctor–patient relationship.
- Basic micro-skills of effective communication.
- Exploring the patient's perspective.
- Making/giving explanations.
- Demonstrating empathy.

It will not focus on the content or structure of the medical history, and will touch only briefly on the basic micro-skills of communication – it is assumed that, as a Foundation doctor, you will already have the basic skills in place.

Key elements of an effective doctor–patient relationship

A recent systematic review of research into the patient–doctor relationship highlighted its complexity and the different ways in which the concept has been described (Ridd et al., 2009). However, the authors identified certain common themes, highlighting how the relationship is enhanced when patients perceive the doctor to be interested, have listened attentively, explained things clearly and involved them in decisions about their care, and when they do not feel hurried. Patients value a longitudinal relationship but not necessarily with an individual doctor, more with doctors as a whole. The depth of the relationship is influenced by several factors, including: perceptions that the doctor cares; the patient's familiarity with the doctor, and vice versa; and trust, which is rooted in their previous experience of encounters with doctors. This results in a virtuous cycle: the better the relationship, the more trust is engendered, and so on.

The findings of the review corroborated those of other authors. For example Stewart et al. in Ontario (2003), in their work on patient-centred care identified caring, compassion and empathy, trust and 'presence' as being key elements of the patient–doctor relationship. Silverman et al. (2005) observe that all the communication skills that underpin the sequential tasks in a clinical encounter such as opening the interview, gathering information, and so on, also contribute to building a strong and effective relationship. However, it is more than just a set of skills and behaviours that can be learnt and reproduced by rote. It must be underpinned by a genuine desire to be involved with the patient at some level.

What's the evidence? Doctor–patient relationship and outcomes

There is overwhelming evidence accumulated over the last 40 plus years linking patient–doctor communication and an effective relationship, with a host of outcomes including:

- psychosocial and emotional health;
- resolution of symptoms (such as pain relief);
- physiological status (such as blood glucose in patients with diabetes);
- adherence to medication;
- quality of life;
- reduction of error;
- fewer complaints.

(See, for example, Stewart et al., 2003 and Silverman et al., 2005.)

Basic micro-skills of effective communication

Attentive listening

Attentive listening is the foundation on which good communication, and in consequence an effective relationship, is built. Rather stating the obvious, it requires the doctor to pay careful attention to both the verbal and the non-verbal elements of the interaction. The key micro-skills of attentive listening include:

- encouraging the patient to talk (without interruption) – using gestures such as nodding, and encouraging noises and statements, for example 'Go on' and 'Uh huh'; echoing – repeating the patient's last words – is a useful technique;

- allowing the patient time to answer questions – not only will this help them tell their story but may also give you time to listen, think and respond;

- non-verbal skills – including body language (e.g. mirroring of the patient's posture, proximity), eye contact, vocal cues (such as tone of voice, rate and pitch of speech), facial expression, and physical contact;

- listening for what's *not* said – either withheld consciously by the patient (e.g. because it's embarrassing) or unconsciously (and may be verbal or non-verbal);

- detecting cues, both verbal and non-verbal – this will be covered below;

- judicious use of silence – to turn a well-known saying on its head, *'Don't just do something – sit there!'*

Any concerns that the patient, if given free reign to talk, will never stop, are largely unfounded. Indeed one study (in an outpatient setting in Switzerland) showed that the 'mean spontaneous talking time' (i.e. how long the patient talked for before they dried up) was only 92 seconds, and 78 per cent of patients had made their initial statement within two minutes (Langewitz et al., 2002).

As much as 75 per cent of the emotional content of an interaction is conveyed through non-verbal channels. Non-verbal communication is a powerful means of helping develop rapport, conveying emotion and, ultimately, helping build relationships. When there is an incongruity between verbal and non-verbal messages, the latter almost always tell the 'true story'. It's not just *what* you say it's how you say it.

Use of questions

Research has shown that doctors often ask too many closed questions, use questions that are too complex (e.g. contain two or more questions within them), ask too many leading questions, and/or don't listen to the patient's answer. As a general rule, it is good practice to start with open questions which encourage the patient to (literally) open up and tell their story. You can then 'drill down' with closed questions to probe and clarify specific facts and issues (adopting a so-called 'open to closed cone'), bearing in mind that closed questions are generally not helpful at promoting discussion or exploring the patient's perspective. Statements can act as questions, and may be less direct, useful when exploring sensitive areas. Compare 'Are you worried about this?' with 'Sometimes when people have symptoms like this they worry about what it might be . . .'; the latter may be more effective at allowing a patient to disclose their fears.

Exploring the patient's perspective

Almost everyone who becomes ill will try to work out what is wrong with them before they ever get to see a doctor. These so-called 'explanatory models' are individual and are shaped by a wide range of factors, including their health beliefs, advice from family and friends, and information from the media and internet. However, more often than doctors seem to realise (largely because they never try to find out), these idiosyncratic explanations are frightening and worrying, pointing, as they often do in the patient's mind, to the possibility of a serious condition.

Unfortunately only a minority of people spontaneously express their ideas, concerns and expectations (ICE), although they will point towards them by offering hints or cues, both verbal and non-verbal. In recognition of this, eliciting ICE has become one of the mantras of modern communication training in recent years. Yet clinical teachers and supervisors often remark how their trainees slavishly elicit ICE, but without any apparent understanding of the purpose or the importance of context and appropriateness, or how to respond when the patient discloses!

Eliciting the patient's ideas, concerns and expectations (ICE)

So why *might* it be important to elicit the patient's ICE? First, we should clarify what is meant by ideas, concerns and expectations:

- *Ideas* are what the patient *thinks* is wrong with them.

- *Concerns* are what the patient *fears* may be wrong with them (not necessarily the same as their ideas).

- *Expectations* are what the patient is expecting from the clinical encounter, and into the future.

Case study 7.1: ICE in action*

Jenny Short was an F2 doctor on nights in the Acute Admissions Unit. She was as busy as ever, with several patients to clerk and a host of tasks pending, her bleep had not stopped since she came on duty and she had not yet managed to have a much-needed cup of tea.

Charles Taylor was a 43-year-old man with a long-standing alcohol problem who was brought in by paramedics having been found slumped in a shop doorway, although he had now regained consciousness. Jenny went to clerk him, feeling irritated, even before she entered the side room, that she was having to 'waste time' on someone who had brought his problems on himself. To make matters worse he was unkempt and smelt strongly of alcohol and body odour.

She started to take a history somewhat curtly, but something about the way he answered her questions made her feel there was more to his story. She adopted a more open and empathic approach, and the story came tumbling out. He had managed successfully to stop drinking for several years, but when his wife left him he was devastated. He left the marital home and had been living on the streets, drinking heavily, for several weeks. However, he had good insight into his problem, but was worried about what damage he had caused, seemed genuinely to want to try to help himself, but, recognising that he would need help, was hoping this would be available. Jenny did not end up spending a huge amount of time listening to him, but came up with some practical suggestions, and when she finally got up to leave Charles thanked her for listening, saying 'I don't know how you can be so understanding to someone like me.'

Discussion

Jenny had overcome her prejudices and had listened to the patient. She had responded to both verbal and non-verbal cues about Charles' ideas, concerns and expectations, and in so doing demonstrated caring and concern, and helped build the relationship. Although she would likely not be involved in his care from now on, indeed may never see him again, she had helped lay the foundation for a future therapeutic relationship.

(*This is based on a true reflective account supplied by Dr Madeleine Long.)

Finding out the patient's ICE potentially serves a number of purposes. In certain settings (such as A&E and general practice) it will usually reveal the *real* (or additional) reasons for consultation, as opposed to what we *assume* to be the reasons(s). It will help you reassure the patient and may prevent unnecessary and time (and resource) wasting diversions into further investigations or referrals. Specifically regarding ideas, it is important to tap into a patient's beliefs – for example, about what might have caused their problem; one of the main factors influencing adherence with treatment is whether or not the patient's beliefs about medicine taking are revealed (Silverman et al., 2005). The need to find out about concerns may seem crashingly obvious, but it is easy to make assumptions about what might be worrying the patient, which, if wrong, might lead to inappropriate and ineffective reassurance. Eliciting expectations is perhaps the area that causes most difficulty, both conceptually and practically. As with other elements of the patient's perspective, this arises partly because doctors make assumptions about expectations, but perhaps also from deeply rooted 'cultural' beliefs that patients have no right to expect anything other than what they get – after all, 'doctor knows best'.

How might we elicit ICE effectively and sensitively? A few simple rules:

- Listen attentively(!).

- Respond to cues, both verbal and non-verbal – this requires both listening *and* observing; response should ideally be at the time the cue is 'offered' or detected, but preferably not right at the start of the encounter.

- Respond to hunches/gut feelings – they're often correct but be aware of your assumptions.

- Offer an empathic statement (see below) – this often leads to disclosure.

- If in doubt, *ask* – sometimes it's better not to beat around the bush, but choice of words is important. A question that is too blunt may cause the person to deny or shrug off a concern.

Verbal cues from patients may take the form of direct statements, expression of feelings, vivid descriptions of symptoms, patients' own attempts to understand what's going on, or loaded statements (Lang et al., 2000). Examples are given in Box 7.1.

Box 7.1 *Examples of verbal cues*

- *Direct statements* – 'I'm a bit concerned'; 'It has me worried'.
- *Expression of feelings* – 'I'm not really worried about this, I just wanted a check-up'; 'My wife's been at me to come and see you about this – she worries about every little thing'. The clue is in the language: worry/worried etc.
- *Symptoms vividly described* – 'Like a red hot needle'; 'I was sobbing with the pain'.
- *Evidence patient has been trying to work it out* – 'Whatever it is I'd like to get to the bottom of it'; 'Something must be causing my . . .'.
- *Loaded questions or statements* – 55-year-old man with poorly controlled Type I DM, 'I've heard that hypos can damage the brain – is that true?'
- *Speech clues* – such as repeatedly mentioning something.
- *Sharing a personal story* – self-evident.

As mentioned above, eliciting expectations is probably the most challenging area. Choice of words is important; compare 'What do you expect me to do?' with 'I have a few ideas about what we might do next, but what about yourself? Do you have anything in mind?' or 'What were you hoping or thinking might happen today?'

Responding to the patients' ideas, concerns and expectations

How should you *respond* when the patient discloses their concerns? Think for a moment how would *you* like a doctor to react to your ideas, concerns and expectations? You would probably want to be taken seriously (however strange your beliefs!)

and would want the doctor to be genuine in their concerns, non-judgemental and empathic. You would probably also want an intelligent and respectful conversation about your expectations. It is important that the doctor does not stifle any emotion (see below), since ventilation of thoughts and feelings can be, in itself, immensely therapeutic. Finally, practical suggestions may be offered, although it is important to remember that doctors don't have to (and indeed can't) fix everything.

In summary, worried, ill or distressed people have a basic need to tell their story and be listened to. Exploring the patients' perspective is more likely to lead to: the *patient* diagnosed, involved and informed, reassured, satisfied and safe; the *doctor*, satisfied, intellectually and emotionally, and less likely to be sued to boot; the *system* guaranteed a safe and satisfied patient, and, hopefully, a doctor who is fulfilled in their work.

Demonstrating empathy

> Patients do not care how much you know until they know how much you care.
>
> (Source unknown)

Patients expect their doctors to be technically competent and knowledgeable, but they also want (and need) doctors who are supportive and emotionally accessible. Empathy (the word derived from Greek roots *em* and *pathos*, literally 'feeling into') is the capacity to imagine what another person is feeling without feeling it yourself, and also to communicate that understanding to them. It is often described as the ability to place oneself in another's shoes, although it does *not* mean 'I *know* how you feel'. Being able to convey empathy is a crucial skill, and has been shown to enhance the doctor–patient relationship, increase both patient and doctor satisfaction, improve diagnostic accuracy, help reduce anxiety and depression, and influence a wide range of outcomes. In the words of one author 'To be understood is intrinsically therapeutic and bridges the isolation of illness' (Spiro, 1992). Absence of empathy is a predisposing factor in most complaints.

Empathy is different from 'sympathy' which means 'suffering with', that is, sharing the other person's distress. Although it may be the natural response to someone else's suffering, an outpouring of sympathy may be unhelpful and may even inhibit the patient out of a wish to spare the doctor. The skills of empathy are not necessarily innate, but they can be learned. However, you don't have to experience the emotions to respond empathically. Further, you don't have to *agree* with the emotion or feelings of the other person.

An empathic response is essentially a two stage process:

- *recognising and acknowledging* the emotions or feelings, through picking up cues from the patient; also through being aware of one's own feelings and responses;

- *responding to* the emotions, by acknowledging them, and inviting further exploration.

The verbal cues may be overt ('I'm really worried about it . . .'), or more subtle hints ('Well, you do worry, don't you?'); the non-verbal cues will usually be manifest in behaviour such as tears or anger.

Empathy can be demonstrated by using simple statements about what you actually observe or can infer from the person's words or behaviour; for example 'You say this has been very worrying' or 'You're obviously upset about how things have turned out'.

Another useful way of thinking about the words you might use is as 'Supportive comments that specifically link the "I" of the doctor and the "you" of the patient' (Silverman et al., 2005). For example '*I* can see that your husband's memory loss has been very difficult for *you* to cope with' or '*I* can understand that it must be frightening for *you* to know the pain might keep coming back'. Some people worry about the form of words they might use without sounding patronising or using platitudes. Reflecting impressions back to the patient may be all that is required. For example, 'Sounds like you were really frightened when you discovered that lump' or 'You're saying that made you very angry'.

It is usually best to respond to the emotion at the time it is recognised, but the level of response must be appropriate.

An empathic encounter is one which leaves the patient with the experience of feeling understood, particularly with regard to the emotional aspects and personal meaning of their illness. There is little convincing evidence that more empathic approaches increase consultation time significantly (Mercer and Reynolds, 2002).

Note, however, that, despite the importance of empathy in the doctor–patient relationship, doctors do need to maintain some professional distance from the suffering and emotions of their patients. This highlights the importance of reflecting on experience, and also of seeking opportunities to discuss, with a trusted colleague or mentor, cases when you have felt uncomfortable or distressed through emotional engagement with the patient (see 'Dealing with emotion', below).

What's the evidence? Empathy

A study of primary care physicians in US (Suchman et al., 1997) showed that patients seldom verbalised emotions directly and spontaneously, but offered cues, verbal and non-verbal (the authors described these as 'windows of opportunity'). However, doctors often ignored cues and continued pursuit of biomedical aspects of the history. Despite this some patients attempted to raise their emotional concerns again (and again . . .) until they finally gave up.

Mercer and colleagues in Glasgow have developed a tool called the Consultation and Relational Empathy Measure for assessing patients' perceptions of empathy during consultations. It is one of several instruments used in primary care to garner levels of patient satisfaction. It comprises a ten-item questionnaire, each item (e.g. doctor seeming genuinely interested in you as a whole person) is graded on a five-point scale from 'Poor' to 'Excellent'; 50 questionnaires are required to give reliable and meaningful results (Mercer et al., 2005).

Giving explanations

One of the most important things doctors do, indeed are expected to do, is to explain things to patients and carers. Doctors need to give information of some kind to patients and/or their carers in most clinical situations, whether on the wards, in out-patients or the GP surgery – see Box 7.2.

Box 7.2 What doctors may have to explain to patients and carers

- Telling people what *might* be wrong.
- Telling people what *is* wrong, which may include breaking bad news.
- Explaining a diagnostic procedure, including the risks.
- Discussing results of investigations.
- Allaying concerns and dealing with misconceptions.
- Discussing treatment options, including their benefits and risks.
- Explaining how to take medication or other treatment regime.
- Explaining why something hasn't worked out, including explaining errors or mistakes.
- Making an apology.
- 'Safety netting', that is, making sure the patient knows what is going to happen or what to do next; for example, what to do if treatment does not work.

Both the quality and quantity of information and the way it is given have been shown to influence a wide range of outcomes, including patients' anxiety and stress levels, satisfaction with care, adherence with treatment, yet many deficiencies have been identified with doctors' explanations. These include problems with both the amount and the type of information provided, the language used by doctors, differences in priorities about what information is important, and the degree of patients' recall and understanding (Silverman et al., 2005). Further, when people are anxious and/or ill, their ability to take on board even simple messages may be impaired. Add to that a sensory impairment, such as deafness, a language barrier, not uncommon in our multi-cultural communities, and a degree of cognitive impairment, increasingly common in the ageing population, and it is easy to see how a doctor's explanation could go completely over the patient's head.

A good explanation is built on trust and good rapport. The latter comes from listening attentively, taking the other person seriously and being empathic.

Explanation will be most effective when:

- the patient's knowledge and understanding is checked at the beginning (particularly important when other professionals have already spoken with them and when breaking bad news);

- the patient's desire for information, both how much they want to know and what information would be helpful, is assessed (not everyone wants to know everything – see below);

- information is broken down into smaller units (so-called 'chunks'), the most important information is given first, and any advice is as specific as possible;

- frequent checks are made on patient understanding (thus the term 'chunking and checking');

- the patient's response is monitored, try scanning for both verbal and non-verbal cues (these may for example indicate that the patient is distressed by or overwhelmed with the information);

- the patient is given the opportunity to ask questions;

- it is appropriately paced and sequenced;

- the patient's knowledge and understanding is checked at the end;

- it somehow connects with the patient's health and illness beliefs.

To aid recall and understanding, various techniques such as 'signposting' (to indicate where the explanation is going and to highlight important facts), repetition and summarising should be used and key (take-home) messages labelled.

Special mention must be made about use of jargon. Jargon may serve three functions: one is absolutely essential, that is, to enable more efficient communication between professionals; the other two are *not* so desirable, namely to conceal vagueness or to hide behind, or to intimidate or control. It is important to remember that the majority of your patients do *not* have a medical degree, thus words such as 'lesion', 'dyspnoea' and 'aetiology' will be meaningless, even to apparently well-educated patients, as will most of the abbreviations and acronyms that abound in medicine. Even apparently straightforward terms such as 'shock', 'anaemia' and 'blood pressure' may have very different lay meanings (and implications). Further, certain words (such as 'syndrome', 'organ failure') may have sinister or frightening connotations or be completely misunderstood (see Case study 7.2). Katherine Whitehorn, the journalist, put it neatly when she said 'Never underestimate the intelligence of your patient, but do not overestimate their knowledge'. Finally, as shown in a recent study, many people are unable to identify the location of major organs such as heart and kidneys, even when they have a relevant medical condition (Weinman et al., 2009). In short, use language and concepts that the patient can understand (see Case study 7.2).

Case study 7.2: (Mis)understanding jargon

Mr Khan was a 67-year-old man from Bangladesh, recently investigated for rectal bleeding. Colonoscopy revealed a single small polyp in the sigmoid colon which was excised; histology showed a benign adenomatous lesion. He attended out-patients for the result, but on being told by the doctor that it was 'only a benign swelling' and that there was thus 'nothing more to be done about it', he became distraught. The doctor was taken aback and asked the nurse to bring his daughter into the consulting room. On further questioning with her help it transpired that Mr Khan thought that 'benign', a word he had heard before in conversations with friends and family but did not fully understand, meant that he had cancer. Further, he thought the doctor was telling him there was no hope, thus that he would die in the near future.

Discussion

The doctor, with the best of intentions, used a word that he assumed everyone would understand, and a phrase that was ambiguous. How often have you witnessed, or have you yourself used, words, whether jargon or not, that the patient clearly misunderstands – it's more common than ever we might think.

Of course not all patients necessarily want information. Evidence suggests this may amount to a sizeable minority (as many as 20 per cent in any given population?), but it is a highly individual preference, is not easy to predict, the influencing factors are complex, and it may change over time and from situation to situation, particularly in relation to bad news (see Chapter 8). The obvious solution is to ask the patient how much they want to know! The challenge is how to inform the majority while being sensitive to the needs of the minority.

Reassuring patients is seen as one of the doctor's major roles. Unfortunately, reassurance, however well intentioned, is often ineffective, and 'the usual culprit for failure to reassure is poor communication' (Fitzpatrick, 1996). If you don't know what that patient needs to be reassured about, and if you reassure them about what you think or guess they're worried about, you will not be able to reassure them, emphasising the importance of eliciting ICE. Furthermore, simply *telling* patients there is nothing wrong may not help, indeed may leave them more anxious than they were to start with (Fitzpatrick, 1996). It is also wrong to falsely reassure a patient; on the whole patients cope better with uncertainty than we might think, and will respect your honesty if you tell them you don't know the answer (see Chapter 8). An especially powerful demonstration of patient-centredness in this circumstance would be to say that, although you don't know the answer, you will try to find out.

As an indication of the kinds of things patients and carers *might* want to know, see the list drawn up by the Patient and Carer Involvement Steering Group of the Royal College of Physicians in Box 7.3.

Box 7.3 Questions patients might want to ask a doctor

- Is there more than one way to treat my condition?
- Do some treatments work better than others?
- What would be the effects of not having any treatment?
- Are any of the suggested treatments likely to cause any problems or side-effects?
- How long will I need the treatment for?
- How long will it be before I feel better?
- Will any of these treatments affect my way of life, e.g. job, driving, hobbies?
- Will I need to take time off work/education?
- Will I need to arrange for someone to look after the people I care for, e.g. my children?
- Do I need to tell other people that I am having this treatment, e.g. work colleagues?
- If I change my mind, can I stop the treatment?
- Do I need to decide today?
- Can I help myself whilst I am having treatment to avoid the problems? (e.g. diet, exercise)
- Where can I get some more information about my condition and the different ways of treating it?
- Who can I contact if I have any more questions after the appointment?

(Royal College of Physicians Patient and Carer
Involvement Steering Group, 2006)

Shared decision-making

The doctor–patient relationship is slowly moving from the historical, paternalistic model ('doctor knows best') to one of partnership (Coulter, 1999). This is both a political and a cultural shift, and the medical profession needs to embrace it rather than carry on as if nothing has changed. Patients increasingly expect to be involved in decisions about their care, and there are clear benefits to all parties when decision-making *is* shared. Yet the reality, somewhat inevitably, is more challenging than the rhetoric. Shared decision-making is the focus of much research at the time of writing (Coulter, 2009).

In terms of what works, key factors include:

- tailored, personalised information;
- patient-held records;

- patient decision aids;

- self-management education + support;

- self-monitoring.

And, of course, an appropriate attitude (willingness to genuinely involve the patient) underpinned by good communication skills, including eliciting and incorporating, as appropriate, the patient's health and illness beliefs and preferences, and communicating risk and benefit. The area of shared decision-making which is arguably the most important, and certainly the most emotionally challenging, is decisions at the end of life; the General Medical Council have produced excellent guidelines on this difficult topic (GMC, 2010b).

Chapter summary

This chapter has:

- covered some of the key elements of communication that contribute to establishing and maintaining a good doctor–patient relationship;

- highlighted that achieving competence and fluency in dealing with some of the more challenging areas (e.g. breaking bad news and dealing with the consequences, handling emotion, etc.) is a lifetime's task;

- reminded you that to a certain extent skills can only be learned through experience and feedback on performance, along with reflection on experience, but there is a strong (and evidence-based!) place for skills rehearsal and practice, particularly in a safer setting than when actually 'on the job';

- suggested that taking every opportunity to get feedback on your communication skills, and to keep them topped up by searching out workshops or courses will make your job a whole lot easier, and will also help your patients.

GOING FURTHER

There is a plethora of books on communication in medicine. All the books referred to in this chapter are excellent sources of information about all aspects of communication: the context, the skills, and the evidence. However, if one could only pick one essential text it would have to be Silverman, J, Kurtz, S and Draper, J (2005) *Skills for Communicating with Patients*, 2nd edition, Oxford: Radcliffe Medical Press. The authors are the creators of the 'Calgary-Cambridge' framework for communication which is increasingly used in both undergraduate and postgraduate training.

Websites

General communication skills

The Online Resource Centre for Clinical Communication Skills at: **www.oup.com/ uk/orc/bin/9780199550463**
Linked with the book by Washer (2009, see references), this website has a range of resources including podcasts, hyperlinked reference list, and website addresses.

The Skills Cascade website at: **www.skillscascade.com/index.html**
This was developed for GP vocational training, its content has general applicability, not least in describing the Calgary-Cambridge framework, also examples of different ways of tackling challenging communication areas.

The patient's perspective

Healthtalkonline is the award-winning website of the DIPEx charity. It is a database of over 2,000 people's experiences of health and illness in a wide range of problems and diseases. The testimonials are available as text, audio or video clips, and are based on qualitative research into patient experiences, led by experts at the University of Oxford. Many of the stories are quite salutory. **www.healthtalkonline.org**

chapter 8

Breaking Bad News and Handling Emotion
John Spencer

Achieving foundation competences

This chapter will help you to begin to meet the following requirements of the *Foundation Programme Curriculum* (2010).

2. Good clinical care: breaking bad news

Competences

- Demonstrates the ability to 'break bad news' to a patient or carer effectively and compassionately, and provides support when necessary.
- Demonstrates ability to communicate complicated or bad news to vulnerable patients, people who are dying, their carers and relatives.

6. Relationship with patients and communication skills: Within a consultation

Competences

- Explains options clearly and checks understanding, encouraging patients with knowledge of their condition to make appropriately informed decisions about their care.
- Deals appropriately with angry or dissatisfied patients.

Knowledge

- How to structure the interview to identify the patient's:

  - concerns/problem list;
  - expectations;
  - understanding;
  - acceptance.

However, *all* the competencies discussed in Chapter 7 in relation to communication and the doctor–patient relationship underpin the ability to break bad news effectively and sensitively.

Chapter overview

By the end of this chapter you should recognise the central importance of the patient–doctor relationship and will be able to:

- break bad news to patients and carers effectively and sensitively and deal more confidently with the consequences;
- handle your own and others' emotion in interactions with patients and their carers;
- call for help with greater confidence.

Breaking bad news

Breaking bad news is an inevitable part of clinical practice. It is never easy or comfortable, but when it is done well the benefits to both the recipient and the giver are manifold. Conversely, when performed insensitively or ineptly, the effects may be long lasting and promote unnecessary suffering. In the words of Rob Buckman, medical oncologist and writer, if we get it right, the patients and their families will never forget us; if we get it wrong, they may never forgive us (Buckman, 1996). There is a strong correlation between a person's perception of the adequacy of information given to them about their problem, and their long-term psychological adjustment. Bad news, however, is a relative concept, and obviously depends on a host of factors related to the patient's life and circumstances. What is devastating to one person may be interpreted differently by another (including by you), sometimes quite unpredictably. This emphasises the importance of using a patient-centred approach, and treating patients individually.

A useful conceptual framework in which to consider bad news is that of 'loss', which is well recognised as a major factor in the aetiology of much psychological illness. The loss need not be loss of life, or even the threat of loss of life. It can be something like loss of a body part, or something more abstract, such as loss of a role (e.g. carer, or physical ability). Whatever, doctors can help to prepare people for the losses that are to come, and breaking bad news (BBN) effectively is one element of this.

In an ideal world, bad news such as a fatal diagnosis, or failure of treatment, should be communicated by a senior clinician. In practice, particularly during unsocial hours, this may be impossible and the task falls to a junior. More often than actually *breaking* bad news, however, as a Foundation doctor you will have to 'pick up the pieces' after bad news has been given. Unfortunately, bad news often cannot be broken gently, but it can be given, and the consequences dealt with, in a sensitive manner and at the individual's pace.

Why might giving bad news be difficult?

There are many possible reasons why giving bad news may be difficult. These include: the 'messenger' feeling responsible and fearing blame; not knowing how best to do it (lack of confidence and/or poor training); inhibition or discomfort due to personal experience of loss; fear of the carer or patient's reaction; uncertainty about prognosis or possible outcomes; not knowing anything about the patient or not having enough information about them, their emotional resources and their limitations; fear of litigation.

These factors can result in one or more of the following responses from doctors: simply not doing it (finding excuses or avoiding the patient), and hoping someone else, for example another colleague or a nurse, will deliver the news; putting it off, for example, by doing more tests; being economical with the truth or using euphemisms, rationalising this by saying they might not be able to handle 'the truth'; avoiding 'cues' or social and emotional issues (one study showed that doctors often used closed questioning and seldom invited discussion when talking with cancer patients); retreating into cold, 'professional' detachment, which may be profoundly damaging to patients and their relatives, and in the long term may affect the doctor's own job satisfaction.

However, there are several practical and logical steps that can be taken when giving bad news. Although all doctors will have their own approach, it is important they: understand what impact the news may have; learn how to deal with the wide range of potential reactions; find ways to avoid feeling blame, and accept that being unable to cure does not mean failure. It is also helpful to have another health professional (e.g. nursing colleague) present when breaking bad news.

What's the evidence? Breaking bad news

A review of the research evidence about breaking bad news in the *Lancet* in 2004 (Fallowfield and Jenkins, 2004) acknowledged that recognition was growing of the need to integrate appropriate training into both undergraduate and postgraduate education. The authors reiterated that 'if communicated badly it (bad news) can cause confusion, long lasting distress, and resentment; if done well, it can assist understanding, acceptance and adjustment'. They also confirmed that skills training is effective, with enduring and beneficial effects, if it follows sound educational principles, is evidence-based, and is suitably assessed. One interesting finding from research is that people seemed to cope better with a traumatic loss when the person breaking the bad news was felt to have shared the emotion in some way – emphasising the importance of empathy.

ACTIVITY 8.1

During your training at medical school you will almost certainly have seen bad news broken both effectively and sensitively, and not so well. Before reading on, think about what factors played a part in influencing the process and outcome.

Several mnemonics and frameworks for 'breaking bad news' have been proposed, all in essence covering similar ground. They include:

- ABCDE – **A**dvance preparation, **B**uild a therapeutic relationship, **C**ommunicate well, **D**eal with patient and family reactions, **E**ncourage and validate emotions (Vandekieft, 2001).

- SPIKES – **S**etting up the interview, assessing the patient's **P**erception, obtaining the patient's **I**nvitation, giving **K**nowledge and information to the patient, addressing the patient's **E**motions with empathy, and **S**trategy and summary (Baille et al., 2000).

Some basic Do's and Don'ts for breaking bad news

Do:

- make sure you have the correct information before you start – this will prevent mistakes, give you more confidence and help you feel more comfortable in saying 'I don't know'.

- create a supportive environment – set aside protected time; make the setting as private as possible; if desired allow family or friends to be present; sit down at the patient's level.

- before, find out what the patient knows already and check the patient's understanding at all stages – this will give you vital information about the gap between their understanding and the medical reality, and whether or not the message is 'getting through'. However, a question at the start such as 'What do you know already' may be too harsh; a gentler 'Have you had any thoughts what your problem might be?'

- assess what the patient wants to know – unless you have an idea what or how much they want to know, you will be unsure if you are giving too much or too little information – direct questions are generally better than 'beating around the bush' in making this assessment.

- give the information in appropriate 'chunks' at an appropriate pace – start with known facts, add to them, continually check understanding, invite questions, take your time; 'warning shots' are often useful, for example allowing the patient to begin to understand that the news is more serious than expected; the appropriate use of silence can give time for the patient to absorb the information; summarise frequently.

- encourage the patient to express their feelings – common responses are: silence, crying, anger and disbelief. Allowing the patient 'space' to express their feelings is vital, as is acknowledging the emotions; don't underestimate the power of touch or silence in these situations.

- explore the patient's concerns and experiences – many factors will influence an individual's concerns for the future, including previous experience, health beliefs, myths and misconceptions etc.). Failure to do this may lead to the concerns remaining undisclosed and the patient preoccupied or overwhelmed by them.

- plan for the future (even if there isn't much of it left) – offer ongoing support and as much reassurance as you honestly are able; patients often feel abandoned and afraid after being given bad news – offering support reduces this fear.

- remember your duty of confidentiality to the patient. This tends to go 'out of the window' as soon as serious or terminal illness is diagnosed; your primary responsibility is to the patient – see below about talking with relatives and carers.

- take great care when indicating prognosis – avoid giving a specific time period, it will only come back to haunt you! You will almost certainly be wrong and the effect on your patient and relatives could be devastating.

Don't:

- use jargon.

- assume anything – for example, about the patient's understanding or their concerns.

- immediately respond to ventilation of feelings with a solution – as before, 'Don't just do something – sit there!'

- try to 'make it all better' – bad news is never good news; on the other hand hope is important, so long as it is realistic hope; there is almost always some reason to be optimistic, if not for survival, then for living until an event such as an anniversary or birth, or for a peaceful, pain-free death.

Giving people the opportunity to discuss concerns and feelings has been found to be therapeutic, leading to more manageable levels of distress. Undisclosed concerns may be the roots of depression and anxiety.

Potential problems when breaking bad news

When a patient asks difficult questions – for example, 'Am I going to die?' – it may reflect a genuine desire to know the facts, but it may also be that the patient is testing the water, perhaps not yet ready for the 'truth', indeed hoping for a 'No, of course not'. In these situations it is always a good idea to reflect the question back to the patient to allow for further exploration. When the patient is apparently unaware of a diagnosis or its implications – firing a warning shot may help – for example, 'The problem is not as simple as we first thought'; using a hierarchy of euphemisms may also be helpful, that is, moving from the least to the most obviously serious scenario (Maguire, 2000); however, one should not force the issue. If a patient is unaware and *doesn't* want information, gentle probing to assess level of denial is prompted, for example, 'Have there been times when you thought things could be more serious?' In contrast, when a patient *is* aware but doesn't want more information, they may tell you outright or offer cues – whichever, their views should be respected.

Although a person may clearly not want any more information, remember that wishes may change over a relatively short time, thus the need to keep checking.

Dealing with emotion

Case study 8.1: Dealing with emotion

It is Monday morning and the Foundation doctor has just started their shift. They are informed that a surgical emergency had not been fully worked up over the weekend, in fact had only been identified shortly before handover. They are on the ward when the patient's partner arrives, and they are given the task of explaining to the partner that the patient needs urgent surgery. Apparently the person has been waiting for a couple of hours for someone talk with them.

As the doctor enters the side-room, the clearly angry and agitated partner says 'Well, about bloody time – someone's bothered to come and tell us what the hell is happening. Where's the doctor? You look like you're on work experience. I hope you are going to at least tell me something positive.'

Think how the doctor might deal with this situation? Then read the next section.

Most doctor–patient encounters have an emotional component, and in certain situations – for example, breaking bad news – emotion lies at the very core. Being able to handle emotion and respond appropriately is an important skill. Empathy is obviously key, and making an empathic gesture lets people know you recognise their distress and are trying to understand it (see Chapter 7). An important strategy is to allow the person to ventilate their feelings, however distressed they are or how distressing the situation; trying to ignore the emotions, stifle or rescue them with platitudes or leaping in with an instant solution is generally unhelpful.

An angry patient or relative is perhaps the most challenging scenario – unfortunately attacks against healthcare personnel are increasing. Anger is often a reaction to the helplessness people may feel when they are ill and passing through a system they don't understand, against a background of fear and anxiety, loss, grief or even guilt. The following tips may be helpful:

- Attend to your own safety first – be aware of where you are in relation to the door, and/or locate a panic button as appropriate; don't allow yourself to get hemmed in; keep a safe distance.

- Try to get the person to sit down, perhaps by offering them a chair – it is harder to continue ranting angrily when you are seated; however, don't sit down yourself until they have done so, as you will be vulnerable if they remain standing.

- Allow them to have their say and try not to interrupt; certainly do not at this stage tell them they are wrong.

- Slow down and lower the tone and pitch of *your* speech – this will usually have the effect of de-escalating the situation.

- Offer empathic statements ('I can see how upset you are') even if that seems to be stating the obvious.

- Offer a *neutral* apology ('I am really sorry this has happened') but try at this stage not to be too specific, until you know the full situation.

- Don't get defensive, and don't tell the person to 'Calm down'.

- Try to avoid mirroring the person's body language, tone of voice.

Doctors have feelings, too, so don't forget, or neglect, your own emotional response to patient encounters (not least when dealing with an angry person). Not only may the patient's emotions affect you and how you behave, but your emotions and feelings can also affect the patient, as well as the consultation process itself (these processes are referred to as transference and counter-transference). Self-awareness is important, and, as stated previously, seeking opportunities to discuss challenging situations with a trusted colleague. Chapters 3 and 18 offer more ideas and strategies about how to develop self-insight and seek help.

Talking with relatives and carers

The patient's family, friends and carers obviously play a vital role in their illness, and communicating with them is an important part of care provision. However, the task of talking with them often falls by default to the Foundation doctor, in terms of 'please tell the relatives' (as if all there was to it was a one-way interaction, with the relative as a passive recipient of information). The same principles for good communication as outlined in Chapter 7 apply as much to relatives and carers as they do to the patient but there are a few specific points to bear in mind when communicating with relatives and carers. Legally the relative, including spouse or other next of kin, has no right to information unless the patient has given their consent; respect for the autonomy of the competent patient must be paramount. The evidence is clear that people are generally opposed to relatives or carers influencing the amount and type of information they receive about their condition, and also wish their consent to be sought before doctors disclose any information to relatives. However, it is important to recognise relatives' need for information and emotional support. It is an area where some discretion, and flexibility – and 'common sense' – must often come to bear. Nonetheless, it can put the doctor in an awkward position which does require tact and negotiation skills; a useful yardstick is to put yourself in the relative's place, or to apply the 'mum test', that is, if this were my mum (dad, sibling, partner, child, granny, etc.) would it be acceptable? What would I want? How would I react?

Some other things need to be borne in mind. Relatives/carers themselves may be trying to cope with, and accept, profound changes in relationship and roles. They may also have specific concerns they may not feel able to share with the patient. A number of factors influence a relative's ability to cope, and thus to support the patient. These include satisfaction with the care provided, an important element of which is the quality of information given, and perceptions about the doctor–patient relationship. As a Foundation doctor you obviously have an important role here. Other factors over which you have relatively *little* influence include the relatives' own emotional and mental state, their resources, psychologically and materially, and the state of their relationship with the patient (beware making any assumptions about other peoples' relationships).

Another common issue is collusion. This occurs when relatives believe that the patient will not be able to cope with the truth (whatever that may be) and ask that they not be told. This will often reflect the relative's *own* discomfort about dealing with bad news, and/or tensions and friction within their relationship, or just family norms, whereby it is difficult or impossible to discuss such issues. Although one must sensitively acknowledge such a request, the general rule should be that if the patient asks about a particular thing such as whether or not they have cancer, and the doctor judges them to be competent, then the issue should be sensitively explored, as described above, and the patient given all the information they appear to want to know. Keeping a record of who has been seen, and told what, when, and by whom is important; it may avoid embarrassing, even distressing discussions in the future, and occasionally may be important when dealing with a complaint.

Calling for help

A key attribute of being a safe and competent professional is being aware of your limitations, thus knowing when to call for help. However, the decision to call for help is not just a technical matter, that is, dependent upon how sick a patient is, or how out of their depth the doctor may feel. A study of the factors influencing junior doctors' decisions about whether and when to call for help showed how complex the process can be (Stewart, 2007). The doctor has to juggle competing and conflicting considerations, including: reluctance to disturb seniors out of hours; concern about what impression they make (calling for help too soon may give the impression of incompetence, delaying calling may make it look like you aren't safe); questions about the usefulness of calling out a senior (would it actually be helpful?); and uncertainties about the different preferences of seniors.

One of the main challenges facing a junior doctor in such situations, and a source of anxiety for some, is how to communicate the request for help in a clear and concise fashion, particularly out of hours and/or when it is anticipated that the senior may be reluctant.

One useful framework for this is SBARR: **S**ituation, **B**ackground, **A**ssessment, **R**ecommendation, **R**eadback. SBARR, which was originally developed in the US, provides a structured approach to communicating important information requiring immediate attention, such as calling for help when a patient's condition deteriorates, or at handover between shifts or between clinical teams, whether the interaction is verbal or written (NHS Institute for Innovation and Improvement, 2010). The tool can be used at any stage of a patient's journey, from the referral letter from the GP to hospital, communication between juniors and seniors, referrals between departments, through to discharge summaries. Chapters 6 and 13 discuss more aspects of communicating with and seeking help from other professionals.

Chapter summary

This chapter has:

- highlighted that achieving competence and fluency in dealing with some of the more challenging areas (e.g. breaking bad news and dealing with the consequences, handling emotion, etc.) is a lifetime's task;

- reminded you that to a certain extent skills can only be learned through experience and reflection on experience, but there is a strong (and evidence-based!) place for skills rehearsal and practice, particularly in a safer setting than when actually 'on the job';

- suggested that taking every opportunity to get feedback on your communication skills, and to keep them topped up by searching out workshops or courses will make your job a whole lot easier, and will also help your patients.

GOING FURTHER

Many of the resources mentioned in Chapter 7 also include sections on breaking bad news.

All the books mentioned in this chapter are excellent sources of information about all aspects of communication: the context, the skills, and the evidence.

Silverman, J, Kurtz, S and Draper, J (2005) *Skills for Communicating with Patients*, 2nd edition, Oxford: Radcliffe Medical Press is a useful comprehensive guide. The authors are the creators of the 'Calgary-Cambridge' framework for communication which is increasingly used in both undergraduate and postgraduate training. It has a section on the Microskills of breaking bad news, as well as other challenging areas.

Another book which focuses specifically on areas of what one might call 'advanced communication', including breaking bad news, dealing with emotion, etc., is Macdonald, E (ed.) (2004) *Difficult Conversations in Medicine*. Oxford: Oxford University Press.

Websites

Pfizers' 'Breaking Bad news' website at **www.breakingbadnews.co.uk**

Healthtalkonline is the award-winning website of the DIPEx charity. It is a database
of over 2,000 people's experiences of health and illness in a wide range of
problems and diseases. The testimonials are available as text, audio or
video clips, and are based on qualitative research into patient experiences,
led by experts at the University of Oxford. Many of the stories are quite
salutory. **www.healthtalkonline.org**

chapter 9

Promoting Health and the Social Context of Healthcare

Lai Fong Chiu and Laura Stroud

Achieving foundation competences

This chapter will help you to meet the following competencies as set out in the *Syllabus and Competences for the Foundation Programme Curriculum* (2010).

10 Health promotion, patient education and public health

Outcome: demonstrates the knowledge, skills, attitudes and behaviours to be able to educate patients effectively.

10.1 Educating patients

Competencies

- Recognises and uses opportunities to prevent disease and promote health.
- Describes the implications of the wider determinants of health.
- Describes the impact of health inequalities on the patient.

Knowledge

- Importance of occupations and wider social and economic factors in disease, and possibilities for rehabilitation.
- Patient education on disease and disease prevention.

10.2 Environmental, biological and lifestyle risk factors

Knowledge

- Risk factors for disease including:

  - social deprivation;
  - health outcome inequalities among ethnic minority communities.

10.5 Epidemiology and screening

Knowledge

- Demographic data collection using ethnicity data to inform health promotion and care planning.

Chapter overview

Clinical medicine often focuses on diagnosing and treating disease, but doctors have an equally important role to play in preventing disease and promoting health and well-being. As qualified doctors working in the NHS, you will operate within the policy framework set by the government of the day, and will be charged with implementing aspects of government policy to improve population health. However, the NHS can do very little by itself to improve population health. In order to realise health improvements, doctors must understand the needs of their local community and work in partnership with other agencies, both statutory and voluntary.

After reading this chapter, you will be able to:

- outline the evidence for health inequalities and the social determinants of health;
- appreciate that there are political discourses that underpin the development of health and health service policy;
- understand how health behaviours and outcomes are affected by the diversity of the patient population;
- explain the importance of community engagement and patient empowerment in health improvement;
- acknowledge the need for the NHS to work in partnership with other agencies to improve and promote health;
- recognise and use opportunities to prevent disease and promote health.

Inequalities in health: the policy context

Clinical medicine is often primarily concerned with diagnosing and treating illness, but doctors should also see the prevention of illness and the promotion of health as an important goal – indeed, according to William J. Mayo, MD:

> The aim of medicine is to prevent disease and prolong life; the ideal of medicine is to eliminate the need for a physician.
>
> (Mayo, 1928)

Historically, the main focus of the NHS has been on treatment of illness rather than prevention. However, in recent years, there has been a recognition that this balance needs to be redressed and that doctors need to take on a much bigger role in promoting health in individuals and improving the health of populations as a whole.

Unfortunately, realising this goal is not straightforward because health is not just a medical issue. There is a convincing weight of evidence that demonstrates a strong association between social deprivation and poor health outcome. This leads to inequalities in health – poor people die sooner.

What's the evidence? Health inequalities

Inequalities in health have been observed ever since statistics have been kept. The first attempt to systematically collect, review and report the evidence in the UK was the Black Report, *Inequalities in Health: Report of a Research Working Group* (DHSS 1980), which showed that a social class gradient existed for almost all causes of mortality and morbidity. At each level of society, those with fewer resources had poorer health outcomes. The gradient in health outcome that Black et al. found is still present today and indeed many subsequent studies suggest that the gap in health outcome between rich and poor is widening. The most recent comprehensive review of the evidence can be found in the report of the Marmot Review team, *Fair Society, Healthy Lives* (Marmot, 2010), which was the culmination of a year-long independent review into health inequalities in England that Professor Sir Michael Marmot was asked to chair by the secretary of state for health. The executive summary of this report states categorically that:

> There is a social gradient in health – the lower a person's social position, the worse his or her health . . . Health inequalities result from social inequalities. Action on health inequalities requires action across all the social determinants of health.
>
> (Marmot, 2010, p9)

For example, according to the report:

> In England, the many people who are currently dying prematurely each year as a result of health inequalities would otherwise have enjoyed, in total, between 1.3 and 2.5 million extra years of life . . . People in poorer areas not only die sooner, but they will also spend more of their shorter lives with a disability . . . even excluding the poorest five per cent and the richest five per cent, the gap in life expectancy between low and high income is six years, and in disability-free life expectancy 13 years.
>
> (Marmot, 2010, p10)

In the face of such evidence, why do health inequalities persist? Clearly, addressing the social determinants of health requires government action, much of which is outside the scope of health services and medical practice. But it also requires political will – for example, the Black Report was commissioned by a Labour government but reported to a newly elected Conservative government that treated the findings of the report with indifference. In the cold economic climate of the early 1980s, the notion of adopting the Black Report's recommendation to spend £2 billion on state welfare programmes to address social inequality was simply not politically acceptable. Essentially, the Conservatives accepted the empirical evidence of health inequalities, but were not persuaded by Black's explanation of the problem or recommended solutions.

How politicians respond to evidence depends on their ideology; in other words, their beliefs about the nature of society. The view that a particular government takes on problems and solutions to health problems will vary. Some governments will not be overly concerned about inequalities in health, provided the overall health of the population improves. Other governments will see the reduction in inequality as a goal in itself, and will focus on narrowing the health gap between the richest and poorest in society.

Governments set out their priorities in White Papers, which define their policies on a whole range of issues, including health. For example, *Choosing Health* (DH, 2004) set out the Labour government's policy on Public Health and Health Improvement, whilst *Equity and Excellence: Liberating the NHS* (DH, 2010a) sets out the Conservative–Liberal Democrat coalition government's plans for reshaping and restructuring the NHS. A change in government will typically lead to a change in priorities and hence policies. Moreover, doctors also need to be aware that their personal response to health policy initiatives is in part determined by their own political beliefs and values.

ACTIVITY 9.1 YOUR POLITICAL COMPASS

Take the political compass test at **www.politicalcompass.org**

What does your political compass tell you about your beliefs about society?

Some governments see health primarily as an individual responsibility, whereas others see health more as a societal issue. The former position has been characterised as 'victim blaming', mainly by those who adopt the opposing position; the latter position is often characterised as the 'nanny state'.

However, there are sound economic reasons for improving health at the population level. Paradoxically, the burden of ill health is not due to a lack of healthcare, and yet most of the resources of the health service are allocated to the treatment of ill health rather than the prevention of ill health. Moreover, the discovery of new diseases and new treatments results in a rising demand for healthcare services, and therefore the costs of providing a healthcare service are likely to spiral out of control unless measures are taken to redress this balance. Finally, health inequalities have a measurable impact on the economy and not just a human cost.

What's the evidence? Preventing disease and reducing health inequalities

The Wanless Report, *Securing Good Health For the Whole Population* (HM Treasury, 2004) concluded that:

> A NHS capable of facilitating a 'fully engaged' population will need to shift its focus from a national sickness service, which treats disease, to a national health service which focuses on preventing it.

The Marmot Review (Marmot, 2010, p9) argues that:

> Action taken to reduce health inequalities will benefit society in many ways. It will have economic benefits in reducing losses from illness associated with health inequalities. These currently account for productivity losses, reduced tax revenue, higher welfare payments and increased treatment costs.

ACTIVITY 9.2 YOUR THOUGHTS ON HEALTH SERVICES

Review Chapter 2 of the Wanless Report, which summarises lessons to be learned from the history of public health policy in England, available at: **http://webarchive. nationalarchives.gov.uk/+/www.dh.gov.uk/en/Publichealth/Healthinequalities/ Healthinequalitiesguidancepublications/DH_066213**

What are your views both for and against the following statement:

> Public health – the promotion of good health and the prevention of disease – should be central to the work of a tax financed NHS. Numerous policy statements and initiatives in the field of public health have not resulted in a rebalancing of policy away from healthcare (a 'national sickness service') to health (a 'national health service'). This will not happen until there is a realignment of incentives in the system to focus on reducing the burden of disease and tackling the key lifestyle and environmental risks (DoH, 2004, p23).

Like the Black Report, the Marmot Review was commissioned by one government but reported to another government – thus, although the aim of the review was 'to propose the most effective evidence-based strategies for reducing health inequalities in England from 2010', there is no guarantee that the new government will implement its recommendations.

ACTIVITY 9.3 RESPONDING TO THE MARMOT REVIEW

Read the Marmot Review, available at **www.marmotreview.org**. What are the key features of the economic case for addressing inequalities in health?

How do you think the Conservative–Liberal Democrat coalition government is likely to respond to the Marmot recommendations?

The NHS is a public service, and thus doctors' work is subject to the priorities of the government. Health policies are subject to economic circumstances, public opinion and political ideology. However, doctors can do much to promote the health of their patients. Marmot identifies six key policy objectives for reducing health inequalities.

- Give every child the best start in life;
- Enable all children, young people and adults to maximise their capabilities and have control over their lives;
- Create fair employment and good work for all;
- Ensure healthy standard of living for all;
- Create and develop healthy and sustainable places and communities;
- Strengthen the role and impact of ill health prevention.

Marmot argues that:

Delivering these policy objectives will require action by central and local government, the NHS, the third and private sectors and community groups. National policies will not work without effective local delivery systems focused on health equity in all policies. . . . Effective local delivery requires effective participatory decision-making at local level. This can only happen by empowering individuals and local communities.

(Marmot, 2010, Executive summary p15)

Inequalities in migrant and minority ethnic groups

Health inequality is not only experienced by low-income groups. The study of health experiences of migrants and minority ethnic groups by epidemiologists has long highlighted the health differentials between ethnic groups and the compounding factor of social class (Balarajan, 1991; Balarajan and Soni Raleigh, 1993; Balarajan and Soni Raleigh, 1995). Over the past two decades, as a result of political conflicts and socio-economic change, Europe has experienced waves of migration both internally and externally. The demographic profiles and social and economic status of migrants in Britain has become increasingly varied and complex (Carbello, 2007). The term 'migrants and minority ethnic' (MME) communities reflects both newcomers and the relatively settled migrant populations in Britain. The experiences of migration and displacement put migrants at risk of poor health due to the unfamiliarity with the health systems and/or simply due to language and cultural differences between themselves and their adopted country. Institutional racism and individually prejudicial practices continue to put the more settled minority ethnic population at risk such as is described in the *Lawrence Report* (McPherson, 1999). Doctors need to recognise that these disadvantages have long-term impacts on health outcomes amongst these population groups.

What's the evidence? Migrants and minority ethnic groups' health status

In 2007, Gill et al. carried out a needs assessment report on the patterns of ill health amongst MME groups in the UK. They found that coronary heart disease is slightly higher in South Asian groups than in the population as a whole, with the Pakistani and Bangladeshi groups having the highest rates. Diabetes is much more common among Afro-Caribbean and South Asian groups, but there is also evidence that it is on the increase among the Chinese and in the White population. Stroke is reported to be an extremely important cause of death among ethnic minorities, being highest in the Afro-Caribbean group and also relatively high in the South Asian and Chinese groups.

Understanding health promotion and the need for patient and community empowerment

Doctors play a key role in disease prevention and facilitating healthier lifestyle changes as every contact with patients is an opportunity for health promotion and disease prevention. You will see that the Foundation competencies include knowledge of a range of risk factors for lifestyle diseases and an expectation that you will know about smoking cessation strategies and the effects of alcohol in particular. However, promoting health requires collaboration between both the public and the private sectors, and the concerted efforts of different organisations and individuals. An understanding of the concept of health promotion and the values and practice that underpin it is important for doctors to carry out their health promotion role effectively.

Health promotion was first defined in the Ottawa Charter in 1986 as 'the process of enabling people to increase control over, and to improve, their health' (World Health Organisation (WHO), 1986, p1).

The Ottawa Charter initiated the health promotion movement around the world. The United Kingdom is the signatory of the Charter and has continued to play a key role in the movement of health promotion by sending policy makers to the successive health promotion conferences.

ACTIVITY 9.4 THE OTTAWA AND BANGKOK CHARTERS

Read the Ottawa Charter (WHO, 1986) and the Bangkok Charter (WHO, 2005) available at:

www.who.int/healthpromotion/conferences/previous/ottawa/en
www.who.int/healthpromotion/conferences/6gchp/bangkok_charter/en

Consider and compare the action areas identified and the recommended strategies. What are the key principles of health promotion? Can you discern any changes as the health promotion concept has passed through time? Where and how do you think doctors can help to realise the goals of health promotion?

After more than a decade, responding to the rapid social, economic, political and technological change brought about by the globalisation process and its impact on inequalities, the World Health Organisation (WHO) has reasserted its goal for health promotion by defining health promotion in the Bangkok Charter as:

the process of enabling people to increase control over their health and its *determinants*, and thereby improve their health. It is a *core function of public health* and contributes to the work of tackling communicable and non-communicable diseases and other threats to health.

(WHO, 2005, p1)

It further reaffirmed its commitment to health for all, and called for actions to build capacity, partnerships and public/private alliances (WHO, 2005). Empowerment, community participation and capacity building are seen as key strategies for achieving structural and systemic change.

Health services should be accessible to all and the care that doctors and other health professionals deliver should be sensitive to diversity, that is, gender, ethnicity, religion, disability, age and/or sexual orientation and regardless of socio-economic status. At the same time, socio-economic status and culture have great potential to influence individuals' health and health-seeking behaviour (Helman, 1994). Effective and compassionate clinical care needs to acknowledge and respect such differences.

From medical school, your own experiences and the discussions and activities above, you know that the task of promoting health is immensely complex. As you become more senior, you will need not only to help patients to avoid risks by facilitating behaviour change but will also work with a range of organisations and agencies to promote healthy public policies and build a supportive environment. Working in support of patients and communities requires an understanding of empowerment. **Patient Empowerment** can be seen as an enabling process by which patients can gain control over their diagnosis, treatment and care whereas **Community Empowerment** enables the community to become an active participant and partner in gaining control over health. Participation and involvement are pivotal to both processes (Chiu, in press).

Information, education and advocacy are essential features of patient empowerment. Although many people now enjoy the benefits of advances in information and communication technology, knowledge gaps and inequalities in access to information still exist. This lack of 'health literacy' impedes access to services and inhibits patients' active participation in their diagnosis, treatment and care.

What's the evidence? Health literacy

The relationship between health literacy and health outcomes was reported by the American Medical Association in 1999. It concluded that patients with low health literacy are likely to have worse health status and an increased risk of hospitalisation. The report recommended that this issue should be addressed beginning with medical education and the improvement of doctors' and patients' communication skills.

Reference: Health literacy: Report on the Council and Scientific Affairs, Ad hoc committee on Health Literacy for the Council on Scientific Affairs, JAMA 1999, 281: 552–557

Facilitating behavioural change through empowering education and communication

Empowering education and communication is important to promote health. Most communication in medical encounters does not stop at eliciting information from patients to reach a correct diagnosis, explain a medical procedure, prescribe a course of treatment or recommend a referral. Doctors are well placed to carry out health education in these encounters to prevent, avoid or minimise further illness through advocating changes of behaviour likely to lead to better long term health outcomes.

A conceptual framework to organise empowering communication

The 'Iceberg' model (Figure 9.1) will help you to examine the relationship between determinants and health outcomes, and to identify health-promoting opportunities that might present themselves through a variety of education and communication in the context of medical practice.

The iceberg (adapted from Travis and Ryan, 2004) is divided into three sections:

1 The top section represents health outcome; it is visible and measurable; for example, hypertension or obesity.

2 The middle section (immediately below the waterline) represents lifestyle; for example, high uptake of alcohol, smoking, over-consumption of fast/processed food, lack of exercise etc.

3 The lower section of the iceberg represents psycho-socio-cultural factors. These are factors involved in determining individuals' health outcomes and they are often more difficult to identify and quantify. They tend to be invisible to doctors who are untrained in health-promoting communication skills.

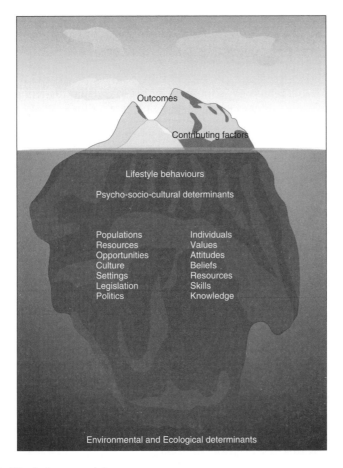

Figure 9.1 The Iceberg model

The bulk of what is taught about communication in medical interviews tends to concentrate on techniques and skills for eliciting information that relates to the middle section; for example, about risky behaviours such as smoking and drinking or about lack of exercise. The resulting health education is often didactic, 'victim blaming' and often ineffective.

So, what kind of health-promoting communication goes beyond the telling and how do doctors empower patients to play an active role in participating in preventing illness and promoting their own health? A detailed description of the communication skills required for health promotion is beyond the scope of this chapter, see the 'Going Further' section for more resources and readings on this topic. However, Activity 9.5 will help you understand how awareness of health determinants can increase your effectiveness in communicating preventative health information to patients.

ACTIVITY 9.5 PATIENT EDUCATION AND COMMUNICATION

From a clinician's perspective, public health information can often be seen as a string of statistics about health outcomes, which appear to have no relevance to individual patients.

Imagine you are a doctor at a diabetes clinic and that someone arrives at your surgery with a history of hypertension or shortness of breath. Using the iceberg as a framework, consider how you might communicate with this patient to help them to reduce their risk.

When this individual stands in front of you, what do you notice about them? You perhaps see someone who is overweight? Whose appearance is florid? Who frequently interrupts their speech to breathe? All this represents the appearance of the iceberg above the water. What do you think might have contributed to the person's health outcome? What kind of question would you ask them or what procedure would you go through to reach your diagnosis?

Apart from carrying out procedures that would lead to a diagnosis and perhaps a course of treatment (information above the waterline), how would you find out what lifestyle factors might have affected your patient?

Would you probe deeper into the possible psycho-socio-cultural factors that might have contributed to their lifestyle?

Some possible questions for probing lifestyle factors:

- What kind of job is s/he doing?

- Might s/he be unemployed?

- Does s/he smoke and has s/he tried to give up smoking?

- How does s/he socialise?

- Does s/he go out a lot, eat processed food or drink a large amount of alcohol?

The kinds of information that might help to understand psycho-socio-cultural factors:

- What kinds of family influences is the individual subject to?

- What values and beliefs about food, smoking, and physical exercise were present in the social environment around the individual when s/he was growing up?

- Where did s/he grow up?

- What social and economic environment is s/he in at present?

The awareness of the way in which these health determinants have impacted and impact on this individual's health will help you to engage with the individual empathetically and sensitively.

Health promotion through community participation

The process of enabling communities to participate in health-promoting activities requires both knowledge of and skills in community engagement. Knowledge includes an understanding of historical and economic factors that affect demographic and spatial characteristics and social and political infrastructure of local communities. This means that local knowledge of work patterns, social interactions and networks, internal and external power relationships of the target communities are fundamental.

Local knowledge is particularly important for engaging new migrant communities and undocumented (illegal) migrants, as, for obvious reasons, little information will be available from official sources for such groups. Local knowledge can be developed through linking and working with community activists in local voluntary sectors.

Case study 9.1: Altogether Better project

The *Altogether Better* (ATB) project is a five-year, £6.8 million, regional (Yorkshire and Humber) collaborative programme funded as part of the Big Lottery Fund's Well-being programme. Its aim is to 'work together [with different sectors and communities] to build capacity to empower communities to improve their health and well being and to reduce health inequalities' (YHPHO presentation 2009). Its programme objectives are to deliver 16 health promotion projects across the region by building partnerships with local communities and governments, primary care trusts, voluntary agencies, universities and other relevant networks. Learning from implementation of the ATB project is shared through a learning network with the expectation that this will impact on regional and national policies on health inequalities, mental health and employment.

Further details: **www.altogetherbetterproject.org.uk**

Recently, community-based participatory interventions (CBPI) such as the Altogether Better project, in which the active participation of communities is the key (including lay and community health educators recruited from target communities), have become an increasingly important strategy to reduce inequalities and promote social justice (Wallerstein, 1992). Doctors are likely to find that support from the communities greatly enhances patient education and health prevention. The community health educator (CHE) model developed to address inequalities of access by MME groups to cancer screening services in the UK in the early 1990s is an established strategy for extending the network of support for patients from services into communities. It has now been adopted by health promotion providers in many guises under names such as 'Health champions', 'Health activists' or 'Health ambassadors'.

The model involves the recruitment of lay members of MME and low-income communities to participate in health promotion activities. Adhering to the critical aspect of health education – 'critical consciousness' – advocated by Paulo Freire (Chiu, 2003), the CHE model challenges traditional didactic health education practice by transforming the form, content and mode of delivery of health promotion programmes. Forming a critical link between the health services and communities, these community health educators, health champions, and volunteers, with their respective language and cultural skills, and armed with their local knowledge can act as advisors, providing information on the cultural beliefs of their respective communities. Programmes conducted in this way are a form of community capacity building (Eng et al., 1997) in which CHEs are invited to collaborate in the planning, design and production of health education curriculum and materials, as well as implementing the health promotion intervention by reaching out to the most vulnerable members of communities (Chiu, 2003). There is a growing body of evidence to suggest that CHEs are effective in reducing inequalities through empowerment and promoting the utilisation of preventive services (Travers, 1997; Lewin et al., 2006).

Last but not least, doctors need to acknowledge that apart from direct health promotion interventions, non-governmental organisations play an important role in tackling the social determinants of health.

ACTIVITY 9.6 WORKING IN PARTNERSHIP WITH OTHER AGENCIES

Identify a non-governmental (voluntary or charity sector) organisation in your local community, and consider how the work of the organisation contributes to the health of the community. Arrange a visit to interview one or more staff about their work:

- Which of the social determinants of health does the organisation address?
- Which statutory organisations support the work of the organisation?
- What difficulties does the organisation face?
- What is the role of the medical profession in supporting the organisation?

Chapter summary

Medical practice in the new century requires doctors not only to perform their traditional curative function, but also to undertake and facilitate health promotion and prevention. However, promoting health is a complex matter. In this chapter, we have:

- illustrated the influences of social determinants of health and how they impact on different population groups;

- highlighted that doctors need to appreciate the wider policy context within which they operate, including health inequalities and population diversity;

- identified that understanding the policy context and the concepts underpinning health promotion will help you to strategise and prioritise your health promotion effort;

- introduced the Iceberg model to help you to conceptualise how you can be more effective in facilitating behaviour change among patients;

- identified that promoting health is not a lone enterprise; it often requires a concerted effort across different sectors and above all the participation and involvement of communities.

GOING FURTHER

Marmot, M and Wilkinson, R (2006) *The Social Determinants of Health*, 2nd edition. Oxford: Oxford University Press.
Chapter 11, 'The social patterning of individual health behaviours: the case of cigarette smoking', is useful as a case study explaining why behaviours such as smoking that are usually held to be subject to individual choice are socially determined, and why doctors need to understand this in order to provide effective interventions to change behaviour.
Chapter 12, 'The social determination of ethnic/racial inequalities in health', expands on the material provided in this chapter.

Naidoo, J and Wills, J (2000). *Health Promotion: Foundations for Practice*. London: Bailliere Tindall.
A good introductory text to the concepts of health promotion

Macdowall, W, Bonell, C and Davies, M (2006). *Health Promotion Practice*. Milton-Keynes: Open University Press.
A companion book of 'Health Promotion Theory', it provides a good range of approaches and practices in health promotion.

part 3

Management, Legal and Ethical Frameworks

chapter 10

Health Management Systems

Stuart Anderson

Achieving foundation competences

This chapter will help you to begin to meet the following requirements of the *Foundation Programme Curriculum* (2010).

7.4 Understands the principles of quality and safety improvement

Competences
F1

- demonstrates knowledge of how and when to report adverse events and 'near misses' to local and, where appropriate, national reporting systems.

F2

- describes opportunities for improving the reliability of care following adverse events or 'near misses'.

11.4 Relevance of outside bodies

Knowledge

- The relevance to professional life of:

  - NHS structure;
  - Medicines and Healthcare products Regulatory Agency (MHRA);
  - National Institute for Health and Clinical Excellence (NICE);
  - European Medicines Agency (EMEA);
  - local authorities.

14.2 Interface with different specialties and with other professionals

Competences

Knowledge

- *Medical Leadership Competency Framework* and *Medical Leadership Competency Curriculum* **www.institute.nhs.uk/building_capability/building_leadership_capability/ project_documents.html**
- Working relationships of:

  - hospital, primary care and mental health services;

- hospital and other agencies (e.g. social services, local authority services, police);
- information transfer from primary to secondary care on admission.

The chapter will also cover some of the leadership and management outcomes set out in the *Compendium of Academic Competencies* published by the UK Foundation Programme Office; the *Medical Leadership Competency Framework* (2010, Academy of Medical Royal Colleges and the NHS Institute for Innovation and Improvement) and *Management for Doctors* (General Medical Council). See also Chapter 14 which covers leadership competencies in more depth.

Chapter overview

Healthcare today is provided by many healthcare professionals working closely together; it is delivered in a variety of facilities with a vast range of equipment. To work effectively these different elements of the system need to work in harmony, and the relationships between them need to be firmly managed. In this chapter we consider the different parts of the healthcare system in the UK, how they are managed and regulated, and what information systems have been developed to help deliver them efficiently and effectively.

After reading this chapter you will be able to:

- describe the key features of health systems;
- list the main types of NHS organisation;
- explain the roles of Special Health Authorities;
- describe regulatory mechanisms operating in the NHS;
- compare the main funding mechanisms in the NHS;
- outline the key NHS information technology programs;
- list the main legislation affecting data security and confidentiality;
- discuss the role of Caldicott Guardians.

Health systems

Health systems are the means by which health programmes and interventions are planned and delivered. In practice, health systems vary greatly between countries. Various methods have been described for categorising them. Roemer (1991) identified five key features which enable a country's health system to be described. These are illustrated in Figure 10.1.

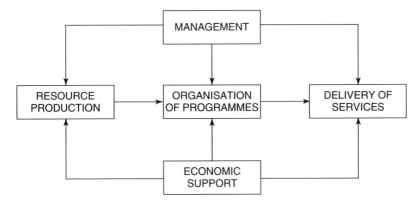

Figure 10.1 The elements of a health system (Mills and Ransom, 2001, cited in
        Roemer, MI, 1991)

Britain's National Health Service (NHS) is an example of a health system. Viewing it as a system is a useful way of describing its key components, for understanding
how they relate to one other and for comparing it with arrangements in other countries. In health systems, the various inputs to health (staff, money, equipment) are
converted into outputs, such as operations, and outcomes, such as improved health.
Roemer's five features are:

- resource production – the inputs of healthcare (trained staff, knowledge required,
  facilities and equipment used, and consumables such as medicines);

- organisation of programmes – who provides the services (whether government
  departments, private providers or voluntary agencies);

- economic support mechanisms – sources of funding (whether taxation, insurance
  or user fees);

- management – the processes involved in planning, administering, regulating and
  monitoring health services;

- delivery of services – the whole range of preventive and curative services provided
  to individuals and populations (these include primary, secondary and tertiary
  services, public health services and services for specific groups and conditions).

Organisational management systems

Organisational management describes the behaviour of organisations and how
they are managed in order to achieve specific goals. Different functions are carried
out at different levels in the organisation, and a wide range of bodies are involved
in healthcare provision. Appropriate arrangements are needed for governance and
regulation. The NHS cannot be viewed as a single coherent organisation; rather, it is

a collection of many inter-related organisations with differing governance and regulatory arrangements. 'The structure of the NHS' describes the main features of these organisations and their relationship to each other.

The structure of the NHS

The NHS has been subject to regular and often radical re-organisation since its foundation in 1948, reflecting the differing philosophies of successive governments and their need to demonstrate that 'the NHS is safe in their hands'. All governments face the enormous challenge of escalating healthcare costs as a result of ageing populations, improved but more expensive technologies including medicines, and increasing public expectations of what medicine can do for them.

The sheer size of the NHS, the fact that it employs around 1.7 million people, and is funded mainly from taxation, means that its management structure is highly bureaucratic in nature. It is characterised by rules and procedures and by a rigid hierarchy of authority relationships. The structure can be illustrated in various ways, including placing the public and patients at its centre as seen in Figure 10.2.

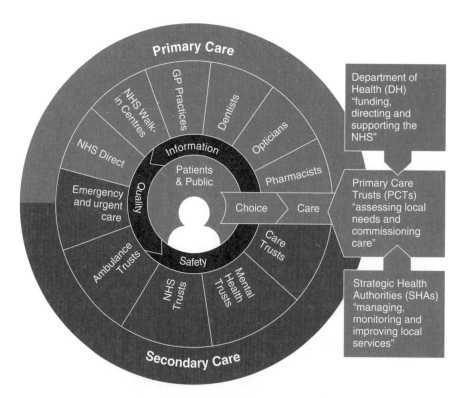

Figure 10.2 The structure of the NHS 2010: The elements of a health system (Figure 11.2 from *National Health Systems of the World, Volume 1: The Countries* by Roemer, MI (1991)). Reproduced by permission of Oxford University Press.

The Department of Health

Ultimate responsibility for the NHS rests with the secretary of state for health, who is accountable to parliament. Members of parliament retain a watchful eye over the NHS and frequently ask questions about it. Aneurin Bevan, the founder of the NHS, referred to this when he said that 'wherever a bedpan is dropped in a ward it reverberates through Whitehall'. The underlying tension between operational and political control remains an important feature of the NHS today.

The Secretary of State heads the Department of Health (DH), which is responsible for funding, directing and supporting the NHS. It does not, however, manage the NHS itself. The DH controls ten strategic health authorities which oversee all NHS activities in England. In turn, each strategic health authority supervises all the NHS trusts in its area. The devolved administrations of Scotland, Wales and Northern Ireland run their local NHS services separately.

Strategic health authorities

Strategic health authorities (SHAs) were created by the government in 2002 to manage the local NHS on behalf of the secretary of state. There were originally 28 SHAs, but on 1 July 2006 this number was reduced to ten. SHAs have four main responsibilities:

- They develop plans for improving health services in their local area.

- They make sure that local health services are of high quality and perform well.

- They identify ways of increasing the capacity of local health services so that more services can be provided.

- They ensure that national priorities (for example, programmes for improving cancer services) are integrated into local health service plans.

SHAs thus provide the principal link between the DH and the NHS at the local level.

Primary care trusts

Primary care trusts (PCTs) provide a range of primary and community services, or commission them from other providers. The main services provided are GP services, dental and optical services, and pharmaceutical services. They provide funding for general practitioners and medical prescriptions and they commission hospital and mental health services from appropriate NHS trusts or from the private sector. There are currently 151 primary care trusts in England, six of which are care trusts.

PCTs are responsible for ensuring that adequate health services for people within their area are available and accessible. These include hospitals, dentists, opticians, mental health services, patient transport (including accident and emergency), screening and pharmacies. They are also responsible for ensuring that health and social care systems work together. PCTs have their own budgets and set their own priorities, although in reality the finance and much of the agenda of PCTs is deter-mined by directives from the SHA or Department of Health. Collectively PCTs are responsible for spending around 80 per cent of the total NHS budget.

Care trusts

Care trusts were introduced in 2002 to provide better-integrated health and social care; they work in both sectors. They are set up when it is felt that a closer relationship between health and social care is needed or would benefit local care services. The NHS and local authorities work together to deliver a range of services including social care, mental health services and primary care services. Only a small number of care trusts currently exist, but more are planned. By combining both NHS and local authority health responsibilities, care trusts are intended to increase continuity of care and sim-plify administration.

Acute trusts

NHS hospitals are managed by trusts. These are either acute or foundation trusts, although there are plans for all trusts to become foundation trusts. Acute trusts are governed by a trust board, which is responsible for ensuring that hospitals provide high-quality healthcare and that they spend their money efficiently. They also decide how the hospital will develop and how services can be improved.

A number of acute trusts are regional or national centres for more specialised care. Others are attached to universities and are involved in the education of health professionals. Acute trusts may also provide services in the community; for example, through health centres, clinics or in people's homes. Acute trusts employ a large proportion of the NHS workforce.

Foundation trusts

Foundation trusts (FTs) are a type of NHS hospital first introduced in April 2004. They are a form of membership organisation known as public benefit corporations. There are three categories of membership: public, patient and staff. Members elect representatives to sit on a council of governors, and are consulted on plans for future development. The council oversees the development of the trust, encourages edu-cational development amongst the workforce, and promotes public health within the services provided by the trust. A board of directors is responsible for day-to-day management, including setting budgets and staff pay.

FTs have been given much more financial and operational freedom than other NHS trusts, and are an example of the government's efforts to de-centralise public services. They are tailored to the needs of the local population. However, foundation trusts remain within the NHS and its performance inspection system. There are cur-rently 130 NHS foundation trusts in England, of which 40 are mental health trusts. Key features are summarised in Box 10.1.

Box 10.1 Key features of foundation trusts

- They are accountable to local people who can become members or governors.
- They have a range of freedoms to decide how to meet their obligations.
- They are able to access capital funds within agreed limits.
- They are able to retain surpluses to help increase investment in local services.
- They have additional flexibilities to recruit and retain staff.
- They are authorised and monitored by Monitor, the independent regulator.
- They are legally bound to work closely with partner organisations.

Mental health trusts

Mental health trusts provide health and social care services for people with mental health problems; there are currently 60 in England. They are commissioned and funded by PCTs, although several of the larger PCTs provide some mental health services themselves. Mental health services are delivered by a variety of providers. Patients usually access the service through their GP or following a stay in hospital.

A wide range of services are provided by mental health trusts. They vary from trust to trust but typically include treatment sessions such as cognitive behavioural therapy, counselling sessions, courses on how to deal with stress, anger, and bereavement, resources such as leaflets, psychotherapy, family support, community drug and alcohol clinics, community mental health houses, and day hospitals and day centres. Patients needing more extensive support can be referred for specialist care, which may involve local authority social services departments, and include specialist services for people with severe mental health problems.

Ambulance trusts

There are 12 ambulance trusts in England, providing emergency access to healthcare. Emergency ambulance calls are prioritised as Category A (immediately life-threatening) or Category B or C emergencies, which are not life-threatening. Emergency control rooms decide what kind of response is needed and whether an ambulance is required. For all three types of emergency, they may send a rapid-response vehicle, crewed by a paramedic. Over the past five years the number of ambulance 999 calls has gone up by a third. The NHS is also responsible for providing transport to get many patients to hospital for treatment.

Special health authorities

Special health authorities (SpHAs) are a type of trust that provide services on behalf of the NHS in England. Unlike other types of trust, they operate nationally rather than serve a specific geographical area. They are a form of 'arm's length body' of the Department of Health, along with executive agencies and non-departmental public bodies (NDPBs).

SpHAs are independent, but can be subject to ministerial direction like other NHS bodies. While they may provide services direct to the public, most are concerned with improving the ability of other parts of the NHS to deliver effective healthcare. There are currently eight organisations that are designated as SpHAs. They are listed in Box 10.2.

Box 10.2 Special health authorities

- National Institute for Health and Clinical Excellence
- National Patient Safety Agency
- National Treatment Agency for Substance Misuse
- NHS Blood and Transplant
- NHS Business Services Authority
- NHS Litigation Authority
- The Health and Social Care Information Centre
- The NHS Institute for Innovation and Improvement

The status of these agencies and authorities is subject to change. A ninth SpHA, the NHS Professionals SpHA, was abolished on 1 April 2010 and its responsibilities transferred to the Secretary of State. The Prescription Pricing Authority was an SpHA until April 2006, when it became part of the NHS Business Services Authority. The Health Protection Agency was originally a Special Health Authority and is currently an independent body.

Plans for restructuring the NHS

In 2010 the coalition government announced that further radical organisational change will occur over the next few years. The White Paper *Equity and Excellence: Liberating the NHS* (DH, 2010a) set out plans to give more power to patients and health professionals. The White Paper describes significant structural change to the NHS.

Among the changes announced, PCTs are to be wholly abolished by 2013, with GPs assuming the commissioning responsibilities they formerly held. The public health aspects of PCT business will be taken on by local councils. Strategic Health Authorities will also be abolished. The government's plans envisage that at least 15 per cent of services will eventually be commissioned from the private or voluntary sectors. The direct services presently provided by PCTs will eventually be commissioned on an 'arm's length' basis.

A further publication, *Liberating the NHS: Report of the Arm's Length Bodies Review* (DoH, 2010b), announced the government's intention to abolish a number of SpHAs and Executive Non-Departmental Public Bodies (ENDPBs). Those scheduled for abolition are:

- Alcohol Education and Research Council;
- NHS Appointments Commission;
- Health Protection Agency;
- National Patient Safety Agency;
- National Treatment Agency for Substance Misuse.

Others are having their functions transferred to other bodies. The functions of the General Social Care Council, for example, are transferring to an enlarged Health Professions Council.

ACTIVITY 10.1 HEALTH PROTECTION AND PATIENT SAFETY

The government has indicated that it proposes to abolish both the Health Protection Agency and the National Patient Safety Agency. Visit the websites of both agencies.

- What are the main activities of each of these bodies?
- Where will these functions to be carried out in future?
- Which activities are to be taken on by other bodies and which are ceasing?
- Which bodies are taking on additional responsibilities for patient safety?

What are the advantages and disadvantages of abolishing national agencies having responsibility for health protection and patient safety?

The evidence on re-organisation

There is now available considerable evidence about the impact that re-organisation has on NHS performance, about what factors are most likely to lead to success, and about what types of re-organisation lead to improved performance. A major review of this evidence was commissioned by the NHS Service Delivery and Organisation (SDO) Research Programme.

What's the evidence? Structural change and NHS performance

- Highly centralised and bureaucratic organisational structures are not associated with high performance, especially in rapidly-changing settings.
- Organisational change needs to be developed from within, not just imposed from outside. Professional engagement and leadership are crucial.

- Frequent reforms have made the NHS unstable, leading to falls in performance in some areas of activity.
- Mergers may not achieve what matters, such as concentrating expertise or removing duplication.
- Occupational 'silos' promote technical change and innovation, but make change management harder.
- The public are reluctant to use 'choice' to influence the services their GPs provide.
- Governments should be cautious about promoting the use of for-profit hospitals.
- No one size fits all: local flexibility in organisational arrangements is important to ensure the best fit to local contexts and cultures, which is what improves performance.

(SDO Briefing Paper, January 2006)

Regulatory systems

Regulation of NHS trusts, staff, and the provision of healthcare is carried out by a number of different bodies, which have themselves been subject to re-organisation. For example, until 31 March 2009 three separate bodies were involved in regulating health and adult social care in England. The Healthcare Commission was responsible for health, the Commission for Social Care Inspection for social care, and the Mental Health Act Commission had monitoring functions with regard to the operation of the Mental Health Act 1983.

Care Quality Commission

The Health and Social Care Act 2008 replaced these three bodies with a single, inte-grated regulator for health and adult social care, the Care Quality Commission. The commission's functions are to assure safety and quality, assess the performance of commissioners and providers, monitor the operation of the Mental Health Act, and ensure that regulation and inspection activity across health and adult social care is coordinated and managed.

Health and social care providers are required to register with the regulator in order to provide services. The Act gives the commission a wide range of enforcement powers along with flexibility on how and when to use them. It can insist on compli-ance with registration requirements, including requirements relating to infection control. It can apply specific conditions for specific risks, such as requiring a ward to be closed until safety requirements are met, and it can suspend services where necessary.

Monitor

Monitor was established in January 2004 to authorise and regulate NHS foundation trusts. It is independent of government and is directly accountable to parliament. It considers applications from NHS trusts seeking foundation status. It considers whether the trust is well governed with appropriate leadership; whether it is financially viable with a sound business plan; and whether it is legally constituted, with a membership that reflects its local community. If satisfied, it authorises the trust to operate as an NHS foundation trust.

Monitor regulates FTs to ensure they comply with their terms of authorisation. These include requirements to operate effectively, efficiently and economically, to meet healthcare targets and national standards, and to cooperate with other NHS organisations. Monitor has powers to intervene if a foundation trust fails in its healthcare standards, or other aspects of its leadership. It also supports the development of NHS foundation trusts, ensuring that they take full advantage of the freedoms and flexibilities available.

The Health Professions' Council

The health professions are regulated by a variety of regulatory bodies: doctors by the General Medical Council, dentists by the General Dental Council, pharmacists by the General Pharmaceutical Council, optometrists and dispensing opticians by the General Optical Council; and nurses by the Nursing and Midwifery Council. A wide range of other health professionals are regulated by the Health Professions' Council.

The Health Professions' Council keeps a register of health professionals who meet standards for training, professional skills, behaviour and health. It was set up to protect the public, and currently regulates 15 health professions. These range from arts therapists and biomedical scientists to operating department practitioners and radiographers. All these professions have at least one professional title that is protected by law. Thus anyone using the title 'physiotherapist' or 'dietitian' must be registered with the council.

Regulating medicines, devices and procedures

A number of bodies are involved in regulating medicines, devices and procedures used in the NHS. These include the Medicines and Healthcare products Regulatory Agency, The European Medicines Agency, and the National Institute for Health and Clinical Excellence.

Medicines and Healthcare Products Regulatory Agency

The Medicines and Healthcare products Regulatory Agency (MHRA) is an executive agency of the Department of Health. It is responsible for regulating medicines including Advanced Therapy Medicinal Products (ATMPs) and medical devices and equipment used in healthcare, and for investigating harmful incidents. It is also responsible for the quality and safety of blood and blood products.

Its main activities are assessing the safety, quality and efficacy of medicines, and authorising their sale or supply in the UK for human use. It also operates post-marketing surveillance and other systems for reporting, investigating and monitoring adverse reactions to medicines, and adverse incidents involving medical devices. It operates a quality surveillance system to sample and test medicines and to address quality defects, monitors the safety and quality of imported unlicensed medicines, and investigates internet sales and counterfeit medicines. It also regulates clinical trials of medicines and medical devices.

'Medical devices' cover products used for the diagnosis, prevention, monitoring or treatment of illness or disability. They include contact lenses and condoms; heart valves and hospital beds; resuscitators and radiotherapy machines; surgical instruments and syringes; wheelchairs and walking frames. ATMPs are either gene therapy medicinal products, somatic cell therapy medicinal products, or tissue-engineered products.

The European Medicines Agency

The European Medicines Agency (EMA) is a decentralised body of the European Union (EU), and is located in London. It is responsible for the scientific evaluation of applications for European marketing authorsations for both human and veterinary medicines developed by pharmaceutical companies for use in the EU. Under the centralised procedure, companies submit a single marketing-authorisation application to the agency. Once granted by the European Commission, a centralised (or 'Community') marketing authorisation is valid in all EU and EEA-EFTA states.

The agency constantly monitors the safety of medicines through a pharmacovigilance network, and takes appropriate actions if adverse drug reaction reports suggest that the benefit–risk balance of a medicine has changed since it was authorised. For veterinary medicines, the agency has the responsibility to establish safe limits for medicinal residues in food of animal origin.

The agency can be considered as the 'hub' of a European medicines network comprising over 40 national competent authorities in 30 EU and EEA-EFTA countries, the European Commission, the European Parliament and a number of other decentralised EU agencies. The agency works closely with its European partners to establish the best possible regulatory system for medicines for Europe and protect the health of its citizens.

The National Institute for Health and Clinical Excellence

The National Institute for Health and Clinical Excellence (NICE) provides guidance, sets quality standards and manages a national database to improve people's health and prevent and treat ill health. NICE makes recommendations to the NHS on new and existing medicines, treatments and procedures, and on treating and caring for people with specific diseases and conditions; and to the NHS, local authorities and other organisations in the public, private, voluntary and community sectors on how to improve people's health and prevent illness and disease.

NICE has an important role in developing and defining standards of healthcare. These indicate when a clinical treatment (or set of procedures) is considered highly effective, cost effective, safe, and a positive patient experience. NICE also oversees the development of the indicators used to determine how GPs are rewarded for providing good quality clinical care and for helping to improve people's health. These indicators are part of the quality and outcomes framework (QOF).

NICE offers advice to pharmaceutical companies and medical device manufacturers on products that may be assessed using its technology appraisal process. Its international division provides advice to other countries on how to ensure that health practices are as effective and cost effective as possible.

Financial management systems

As providers of care, health professionals are responsible for committing large sums of money. They not only order diagnostic tests and prescribe medicines but also use theatre and other resources, as well as the time of support staff. In 2010 the total sum allocated for healthcare for the United Kingdom was £119.5 billion. Around 90 per cent of this sum comes from public funding; of this about 78 per cent comes from general taxation and the rest from National Insurance contributions. Of the 10 per cent that comes from other sources, around 2 per cent comes from patient charges, about 5 per cent from capital refunds such as land sales, and the remainder from miscellaneous sources.

Clinicians therefore need to have an understanding of the funding and purchasing of healthcare. In the NHS a number of different mechanisms are used to distribute funds to healthcare providers. In primary care, contracts for doctors, dentists and pharmacists are negotiated nationally but usually allow room for local flexibility. The contracts are held with local PCTs. For secondary care, SHAs fund providers through an assortment of mechanisms which take account of population needs and level of demand.

Payment by results (PbR)

PbR is a method of funding NHS activity which was first used in England in 2003/04. It replaced a system where provider funding was reliant principally on historic budgets and the negotiating skills of individual managers. Its aim is to provide a transparent, rule-based system for the payment of healthcare providers. It seeks to reward efficiency, support patient choice and encourage productivity.

Payments are linked to activity and adjusted for case-mix. PbR is based on a system of nationally set prices or tariffs. For inpatient care, PbR uses Healthcare Resource Groups (HRGs) which are a unit of payment based on individual patient episodes. Groups of patients having similar diagnoses are grouped together. For outpatients, hospitals are paid for attendances. Each specialty has two groups of activity, first and follow-up appointment, each with its own tariff. The tariff for each HRG and outpatient code is based on the average cost of treatment. Costs are reported yearly as part of the annual reference cost exercise.

ACTIVITY 10.2 IS PAYMENT BY RESULTS THE ANSWER?

Read about PbR on the following website: **www.dh.gov.uk/en/Managingyour organisation/NHSFinancialReforms/index.htm**

- What clinical services are now covered by the PbR system?
- What are the advantages of a PbR system over an historic budget system?
- What are the disadvantages of a PbR system?

Is any account taken in PbR of the fact that it is more expensive to provide services in some parts of the country than in others?

Quality and outcomes framework (QOF)

The QOF is a system for the performance management and payment of GPs in the NHS in England, Wales and Scotland. It was introduced as part of the general medical services contract in April 2004, replacing a variety of fee arrangements. It was intended to improve the quality of general practice and was part of an effort to solve a shortage of GPs. QOF rewards GPs for implementing 'good practice' in their surgeries.

Practices can accumulate up to 1050 QOF points, depending on level of achievement for each of 146 indicators. The criteria are grouped into four domains: clinical, organisational, patient experience and additional services. At the end of the financial year the total number of points achieved is collated by QMAS or another system (see below), which then converts the points into a payment for the surgery. The formula includes numbers of patients, including numbers diagnosed with certain common chronic illnesses.

Practice-based commissioning (PBC)

PBC is a process by which responsibility for commissioning services is devolved from PCTs to local GP practices. Under PBC, practices are given a commissioning budget which they use to provide services. This involves identifying patient needs, designing effective and appropriate health service responses, and allocating resources against competing service priorities. PBC is intended to give local clinicians greater control over resources. GPs, nurses and other primary care professionals are in the prime position to translate patient needs into redesigned services. PCTs are the budget holders and have overall accountability for healthcare commissioning. Practice-based commissioners work closely with PCTs and secondary care clinicians, and lead work on deciding clinical outcomes. They also play a key supporting role to PCTs by providing feedback on provider performance.

Financial control

Detailed cost records are essential if costs are to be controlled. Records are needed in management accounting to assist internal management decisions in day-to-day operations and in the planning and controlling of activity; and in financial accounting to enable the organisation to produce financial statements in the format required by government or supervisory bodies, and to provide people outside the organisation with detailed and accurate information about the financial situation.

Health professionals are ideally place to identify ways in which cost savings might be made and where efficiencies can be found. These need to be encouraged, but not all apparent savings will be deliverable in practice. There are a number of financial pitfalls to avoid, such as the overheads trap. Read case study 10.1 for an example of how the overheads trap works in practice.

Case study 10.1: In-house or out-source? The overheads trap

The Windward Hospital has a laundry that provides services for all hospital wards. However, a newly launched commercial laundry has approached several budget managers with a view to providing a cost-effective service of equal quality to that provided by the hospital. The costs for the hospital's laundry are:

Direct costs:	£000s
Staff costs	50
Consumables	5
Overheads and cross charges inwards:	
Capital charges	3
Energy	10
Housekeeping	10
Maintenance	5
Administration	10
Total costs:	93

During the year the laundry processed 150,000 items, 18,000 of which were charged to the surgical ward on a standard cost basis. The budgets for the coming year have already been set on the basis that there will be no change in the laundry budget over the previous year and no change in the surgical ward's laundry requirements. However, the manager of the surgical ward thinks that buying in laundry services may save money.

You are asked to examine the figures. The commercial laundry quotes £50 per 100 items for 18,000 items over a one-year period, or £0.50 per item. The standard cost per item for the in-house laundry is calculated by dividing each cost by the planned activity. For staff this is £0.33, for consumables £0.03, and for overheads £0.25, making a total of £0.61 per item.

For 18,000 items the cost to the surgical ward would be £10,980 using the in-house laundry, but £9,000 using the commercial one, an apparent saving of £1,980. But the cross-charge income of the in-house laundry would be reduced by £10,980. Although there would be some reduction in use of consumables, the in-house laundry would have to increase its cross charges to the other departments.

Although there is an apparent saving of £1,980 to the surgical ward, the actual cost to the hospital if it bought its laundry service commercially is £10,980 less £540 for consumables. Only variable costs are saved; fixed costs are still incurred. This is the overheads trap.

(Adapted from Gruen and Howarth, 2005, pp103–5)

Code of conduct for NHS managers

A code of conduct for NHS managers was produced as part of the response to the Kennedy Report on baby deaths at Bristol Royal Infirmary in 2001. The code sets out core standards of conduct expected of NHS managers. It has two main functions:

- to guide NHS managers and employing health bodies in the work they do and the decisions and choices they have to make;

- to reassure the public that these important decisions are being made against a background of professional standards and accountability.

The code operates in a complex environment. NHS managers work in very public and demanding situations. The management of the NHS calls for difficult decisions and complicated choices. Managers and clinicians often have differing priorities; the interests of individual patients have to be balanced with the interests of groups of patients and of the community as a whole. A balance also has to be maintained between national and local priorities. The code applies to all managers in the NHS.

Information management systems

Extensive use of information technology is essential for effective healthcare delivery and performance management, and the NHS has devoted massive resources to it. A separate field of study has emerged around the subject, and the Department of Health has established a separate body to take forward the development of its IT programme. Health informatics (also called healthcare informatics or medical informatics) is the intersection of information science, computer science, and healthcare. It deals with the resources, devices, and methods required to optimise the acquisition, storage, retrieval, and use of information in health and biomedicine.

Health informatics tools include not only computers but also clinical guidelines, formal medical terminologies, and information and communication systems. It is applied in many areas of healthcare including nursing, clinical care, dentistry, pharmacy and public health, as well as biomedical research.

NHS Connecting for Health

NHS Connecting for Health was established in April 2005 as an agency of the Department of Health, replacing the former NHS Information Authority. Its purpose is to support the NHS in providing better, safer care, by delivering computer systems and services that improve how patient information is stored and accessed.

The NHS National Programme for IT (NPfIT)

NPfITis the Department of Health initiative designed to provide for the NHS in England a range of IT initiatives including a single, centrally mandated electronic care record for patients, and a system to connect 40,000 general practitioners to over 300 hospitals, providing secure and audited access to these records by authorised health professionals. Connecting for Health is responsible for delivering it.

The national network for the NHS (N3)

N3 was established to provide a reliable, supporting IT infrastructure, along with networking services and sufficient, secure connectivity and broadband capacity to meet current and future NHS IT needs. It replaced NHSnet, the previous private NHS communications network in England. N3 underpins and enables the delivery of new IT systems and services for the NHS. These applications all require reliable bandwidth in excess of that provided by NHSnet. N3 provides connectivity to all NHS organisations in England, as well as those non-NHS sites providing NHS care. Its function is to ensure a reliable service at every site where NHS services are delivered or managed.

N3 is delivered by NHS Connecting for Health. An N3 Service Provider (N3SP) has been appointed to take responsibility for integrating and managing the service. The N3 service has been procured from a number of subcontractors to ensure value for money; the N3SP brings together the separate elements into a complete and seamless end-to-end network, whilst ensuring flexibility and best value for the NHS. The N3SP also manages the network, dealing with, for example, fault reporting and customer relationship management.

Choose and Book

Choose and Book is an electronic appointments booking service which gives patients a choice of place, date and time for their first outpatient appointment in a hospital or clinic. It is up and running and reached 20 million referrals in March 2010. It allows patients who have been referred to a specialist by their GP to book, change or cancel their appointment online or by phone. They require an appointment reference number and a password.

Choose and Book shows the GP which hospitals or clinics are available to provide treatment. It may be possible to book the appointment before the patient leaves the surgery, although they may be given an appointment request letter and book the appointment later. Although the vast majority of appointments can be booked in this way, Choose and Book is not yet universal, as not all hospital computers are linked to it. In some cases, patients have to telephone their chosen hospital directly to make an appointment.

Picture Archiving and Communications Systems (PACS)

PACS are medical imaging software that enable images such as X-rays and scans to be stored electronically and viewed on-screen, creating a near filmless process and improved diagnosis methods. PACS consist of four major components: the imaging modalities such as CT and MRI, a secure network for the transmission of patient information, workstations for interpreting and reviewing images, and archives for the storage and retrieval of images and reports.

PACS replace hard-copy-based means of managing medical images such as film archives, and with the decreasing price of digital storage, it provides a cost and space advantage over film archives in addition to instant access to images at the same institution. It also allows remote access, providing capabilities of off-site viewing and reporting to facilitate distance education and tele-diagnosis. It provides the electronic platform for radiology images to interface with other information systems such as hospital information systems and electronic medical records. Finally, it is used by radiology personnel to manage workflow.

Electronic Prescription Service (EPS)

EPS is the NHS system for the electronic transmission of prescription information. E-Prescribing systems enable medications (and other prescribed therapies) to be managed electronically at every stage, from prescribing through to supply and administration. They replace paper prescriptions that would otherwise be carried to the pharmacy by the patient or be at the patient's bedside. They are claimed to improve patient safety by reducing the possibility of prescribing and administration errors.

E-Prescribing systems support the whole medicines use process: computerised entry of prescriptions; computerised links between hospital wards/departments and pharmacies; and, ultimately, links to other elements of patients' individual care records. Knowledge support is available with immediate access to medicines information such as the British National Formulary; decision support, aiding the choice of medicines and other therapies, with alerts such as drug interactions; and a robust audit trail for the entire medicines use process.

GP2GP

GP2GP is the national system that enables patients' electronic health records to be transferred directly and securely from one GP practice to another. It is part of the National Programme for IT. One million electronic health records had been transferred using the GP2GP service by February 2010.

Over 5,000 GP practices across the country can now use the GP2GP service, allowing patients' electronic health records to be transferred reliably and securely between practices in a matter of moments, resulting in increased patient safety and continuity of care. This number will grow as more GP practices are enabled and a greater number of systems become available.

The quality management and analysis system (QMAS)

QMAS is a national IT system for performance management in primary care QMAS). It gives GP practices and Primary Care Trusts (PCTs) objective evidence and feedback on the quality of care delivered to patients. It supports the Quality and Outcomes (QOF) element of the GP contract and has been in operation since 2004. QMAS shows how well each practice is doing, measured against national QOF achievement targets. It allows practices to analyse the data they collect about the number of services and quality of care they deliver, such as the services provided to patients with the chronic diseases included in QOF.

Access to the system is also provided to PCTs so that practices and PCTs can share information throughout the year. As practices are rewarded financially according to the quality of care provided, the payment rules that underpin the GMS Contract need to be implemented consistently across all systems and all practices in England. QMAS ensures that this is achieved.

NHSmail

NHSmail is a secure, web-based email service developed for the NHS in England and Scotland. It is designed to comprise an integrated and secure email, diary and

directory system for NHS employees, and offers access from any networked computer as well as from mobile devices. NHSmail provides a secure, encrypted means of
exchanging information.

The NHSmail system uses a customised version of Microsoft Exchange (2007)
and thus may be accessed by Microsoft Outlook on Windows or Microsoft Entou-
rage on Apple OS X. Other systems may also be used. Mobile devices which support
Exchange email and calendar may be configured to use NHSmail email and calendar functions, either with native capability or by installing third-party software.
NHSmail also offers an SMS gateway, allowing users to send SMS messages, and a
number of mobile devices are also supported.

ACTIVITY 10.3 PROGRESS WITH IT

Computing developments are moving forward very rapidly in the NHS. Go to the
connecting for health website at **www.connectingforhealth.nhs.uk**.

- What changes have been made to the services listed above?
- What other IT services and systems are now available?
- What arrangements do these services replace?
- Who is responsible for providing them?
- What are the consequences for patients?
- What do doctors need to do as a result?

Data management systems

A wide range of legislation relates to the management of data; this includes the European Data Protection Directive, the Data Protection Act 1998, the Freedom of Information Act 2000, and the Computer Misuse Act 1992. These are now briefly outlined.

European Data Protection Directive

The European Data Protection Directive is officially Directive 95/46/EC on the protection of individuals with regard to the processing of personal data and on the free
movement of such data. The directive was implemented in 1995 by the European Commission, and is an important component of European Union (EU) privacy and human
rights law. The directive regulates the processing of personal data within the EU.

Personal data are defined as 'any information relating to an identified or identifiable natural person' (data subject). An 'identifiable person' is one who can be identified, directly or indirectly, by reference to an identification number or to one or more
factors specific to his physical, physiological, mental, economic, cultural or social
identity. This definition is very broad. Data are 'personal data' when someone is able
to link the information to a person, even if the person holding the data cannot make

the link. Examples of personal data include address, credit card number, bank statements, or criminal record.

Data Protection Act 1998 (DPA)

The DPA is a United Kingdom Act of Parliament which defines UK law on the processing of data on identifiable living people. It is the main piece of legislation that governs the protection of personal data in the UK. Although the Act itself does not mention privacy, it was enacted to bring UK law into line with the European Directive of 1995 which required member states to protect people's fundamental rights and freedoms and in particular their right to privacy with respect to the processing of personal data.

In practice it provides a way for individuals to control information about themselves. Anyone holding personal data for other than domestic purposes is legally obliged to comply with this Act, subject to some exemptions. The Act defines eight data protection principles.

Freedom of Information Act 2000

The Freedom of Information Act 2000 applies in the United Kingdom at the national level. It introduced a public 'right to know' in relation to public bodies. The full provisions of the Act came into force on 1 January 2005. The Act led to the renaming of the Data Protection Commissioner (set up to administer the Data Protection Act) as the Information Commissioner, whose office oversees the operation of the Act.

A second freedom of information law is in existence in the UK, the Freedom of Information (Scotland) Act 2002. This was passed by the Scottish parliament in 2002, to cover public bodies over which the Holyrood parliament, rather than Westminster, has jurisdiction. For these institutions, it fulfils the same purpose as the 2000 Act.

Computer Misuse Act 1990

The Computer Misuse Act 1990 is relevant to electronic records in that it creates three offences of unlawfully gaining access to computer programs: the unauthorised access to computer material; unauthorised access with intent to commit or cause commission of further offences; and unauthorised modification of computer material.

Access is defined in the Act as altering or erasing the computer program or data; copying or moving the program or data; using the program or data; or outputting the program or data from the computer in which it is held. Unlawful access is committed if the individual intentionally gains access, knowing he is not entitled to do so, and aware he does not have consent to gain access. The 'further offence' applies if unauthorised access is carried out with intent to commit or cause an offence. The 'modification' offence applies if an individual carries out any act causing unlawful modification of computer material.

Caldicott Guardians

A number of strategies have been developed to address the issues of patient confidentiality. One of these is the nomination of a Caldicott Guardian. A Caldicott Guardian is a senior person responsible for protecting the confidentiality of patient and service-user information and enabling appropriate information-sharing. Each NHS and social care organisation that has access to patient records is required to have one. It therefore includes acute trusts, ambulance trusts, mental health trusts, PCTs, SHAs, and SpHAs such as NHS Direct.

The role of the guardian is to ensure that NHS organisations, councils with social services responsibilities, and partner organisations satisfy the highest practical standards for handling patient identifiable information. The guardian acts as the 'conscience' of the organisation, actively supporting work to enable information-sharing where it is appropriate, and advising on options for lawful and ethical processing of information.

The guardian also has a strategic role, which involves representing and championing information governance requirements and issues at board or management team level. The role is particularly important in relation to the implementation of NPfIT and the development of Electronic Social Care Records and Common Assessment Frameworks.

Chapter summary

In this chapter we have considered:

- the role of the Department of Health, SHAs, PCTs and other parts of the NHS;

- the function of arm's length bodies including special health authorities;

- mechanism for regulating healthcare standards, health organisations and health professionals;

- financial management mechanisms in the NHS including Payment by Results, Practice Based Commissioning and the Quality and Outcomes Framework;

- the key IT programmes developed by Connecting for Health;

- issues of data security and confidentiality;

- the role of the Caldicott Guardian.

GOING FURTHER

Black, N and Gruen, R (2005) *Understanding Health Services*. Maidenhead, Berks:
Open University Press.
A more detailed discussion of the main topics within financial management in
healthcare.

Gruen, R and Howarth, A (2005) *Financial Management in Health Services*. Maidenhead, Berks: Open University Press.
A general introduction to health services at the individual, organisational and
national levels.

Wager, KA, Lee, FW and Glaser, JP (2009) *Healthcare Information Systems: A Practical
Approach for Healthcare Management*. San Francisco, CA: Jossey-Bass.
A general introduction to managing healthcare information.

Iles, V (2005) *Really Managing Healthcare,* 2nd edition. Maidenhead, Berks: Open
University Press.
A practical guide to managing people, money and change in healthcare.

chapter 11

Principles of Medical Ethics and Confidentiality

Dominic Bell

Achieving foundation competences

This chapter will help you begin to meet the following requirements of the *Foundation Programme Curriculum* (2010):

Competences
F1 and F2

- Describes and demonstrates an understanding of the main principles of medical ethics, including autonomy, justice, beneficence, non-maleficence and confidentiality as they apply to medical practice.
- Ensures privacy when discussing sensitive issues.
- Uses and shares clinical information appropriately or seeks advice when uncertain (see Professionalism: Behaviour in the workplace).
- Seeks timely advice where patient abuse is suspected, while respecting confidentiality.
- Modifies patients' management plans in accordance with the principles of patients' best interests, autonomy and rights.

Knowledge

- GMC guidance on specific ethical issues and guidance on consent.
- Principles of patients' best interests.
- Ethical principles and legal framework in relation to autonomy, medical research and human rights (including advance directives).
- Strategies to ensure confidentiality.
- Functions of Caldicott Guardians.
- Limits to confidentiality.
- Data Protection Act/Freedom of Information provisions.

Chapter overview

The law offers a guide to doctors on how we should act in certain circumstances. However, determining what is the *right* thing to do in your work often requires something different from an encyclopaedic knowledge of medical law or professional guidelines. This is when an understanding of the ethical principles that apply to medical practice and the framework in which issues can be explored in a consistent and reasoned manner is useful. Although the global and political elements of ethical debates may sometimes seem remote and irrelevant, almost every aspect of our professional responsibilities has a significant ethical undertone.

After reading this chapter, you will be able to:

- describe some of the key issues in medical ethics and relate these to your own professional practice;
- apply ethical concepts to your own practice in the light of legal rules and your own beliefs;
- discriminate between different standpoints on ethical issues and understand from where these have been derived.

Applicability of ethics

ACTIVITY 11.1 APPLICABILITY OF ETHICS

Medical ethics is often linked with 'dilemmas' such as euthanasia and abortion. However, it is much wider than this. Look at the next three scenarios and think how you would act in these circumstances.

- What would you do if you were asked to perform a procedure you were not fully trained in? But you really want to practise it and are sure you can do it adequately.
- A close friend asks you to take something from work – there are lots of them and they are cheap.
- A colleague's behaviour at work has been erratic and you are concerned about patient care. Would it make a difference if the colleague was a peer or the consultant?

As you know, making ethical decisions often leads us into grey areas where we need to consider our own moral position and beliefs, what the law tells us and what professional guidance says.

If ethics, as an integral component of medical practice, is to be valued by practitioners, patients, the public, politicians and the law, it needs to be clearly and consistently defined. This revolves around the rational evaluation of core and often competing ethical principles, the structure of ethical advisory bodies and the process by which a position is reached on a particular subject.

Any ethical argument therefore needs to review the neutrality of the authors, the goals of the exercise (explicit or otherwise), and the process by which the argument was derived. This highlights that ethics has to go beyond the individual religious or secular beliefs of practitioners, even if the underlying argument is patient-orientated such as 'respect for autonomy'. For example, a patient may want their life ended and a practitioner may feel sympathetic to their request, but to proceed in the clear knowledge of the position at law would demonstrate lack of awareness of one's responsibilities to the patient, public and the profession, and risk the reputation, livelihood and liberty of the practitioner.

Our professional responsibilities are based on the nature of our relationship with patients, their need for trust and confidence, and the unwritten rule that we must never jeopardise that trust. The areas in which trust applies include competence and performance, the exercise of professional judgement, confidentiality and conduct. Working within limits of competence is a specified condition of registration, whilst professional judgement incorporates competence and the ethical principles of beneficence and non-maleficence as discussed below. The more complex areas are confidentiality and conduct.

Respect for autonomy

The principle of autonomy is underpinned by a fundamental respect for human agency and rights, the drive towards more patient empowerment and the freedom to make independent, informed choices. For doctors, respecting autonomy can be problematic when it comes with the associated loss of 'benign paternalism', an issue which requires the highest level of ethical debate. Not every patient has the ability or the inclination to process an abundance of medical information when reaching a decision and the quality of decision-making on the part of the patient may be compromised by the pressure to reach a decision, in isolation, under the principle of respect for autonomy. Whilst paternalism has a negative connotation within regulatory bodies and amongst media commentators, a significant proportion of the population wish to be assisted in decision-making by their medical practitioner and trust their experience and expertise. It would be detrimental to both profession and public if this vocational privilege were to be lost.

Beneficence and non-maleficence

'Respect for autonomy' introduces the accompanying concepts of beneficence (doing good) and non-maleficence (doing no harm), the principles consolidated by Beauchamp and Childress (2001) and now seemingly universally accepted. The concepts should be applied in every healthcare decision in reaching informed consent, or when decision-making has to be taken for a patient lacking capacity. There is absolute harmony between these principles and those utilised when reaching a 'best interests' determination under the Mental Capacity Act, whereby a balance sheet of the benefits and potential detriment of any proposed course of action is drawn up. This should therefore be a sterile area for debate, but most doctors would concede that a range of opinion will usually be available on what is good for a particular patient and different medical specialties may consistently present polarised views.

For example, an oncologist may recommend radiotherapy or chemotherapy, or a surgeon an operation, as opposed to a general practitioner or palliative medicine clinician, who may put more weight on the adverse consequences of such interventions for the limited advantages in survival and recommend symptomatic relief only. The law and all professional guidance emphasises that best interests go beyond medical best interests and accommodate the patient's values and beliefs, including religious and secular, which must be explored. There is always an ethical challenge therefore, and every practitioner should be able to divorce themselves from their own specialty interests and values when reaching such a decision.

Justice

The fourth fundamental principle, that of justice, invariably triggers maximal ethical debate, professional divisions, adverse media commentary, and legal challenges. The concept of ensuring that the benefits, risks and costs of healthcare are distributed fairly, and that patients with similar conditions should be treated identically regardless of geographical area, cultural background or lifestyle, stimulates endless debate. These issues are particularly pertinent at a time of global recession, forcing choice between, for example, expensive chemotherapy to briefly extend the lives of a few, and vaccination programmes to prevent less debilitating illness in the many or investing either in reactive secondary care in hospitals or in public-health strategies to prevent the development or progression of disease in the community. This also triggers analysis of the healthcare benefits of increasing funding to social care and education rather than to healthcare itself.

Although some section of the population will always be disadvantaged by these decisions, decisions must be taken primarily on utilitarian grounds to maximise overall benefit from public investment. Utilitarianism is therefore an appropriate ethical principle in some circumstances, but different criteria would be applied to this category of decision-making if considering ethical defensibility. Any decision made by a multitude of advisory and authoritative bodies must be transparent, free from any conflict-of-interest, and open to challenge or judicial review on the criteria that have been used to make the decision and how the criteria are applied in practice.

Confidentiality

The duty of confidentiality is considered so fundamental to individual and public confidence as to warrant specific professional guidelines and be enshrined in law as set out in Chapter 12. Unless confident that information given to a doctor will only be used to enable the correct diagnosis to be reached and for the optimal treatment to be administered, the individual patient may either not attend or may withhold information and thereby compromise their own well-being and that of others.

Regardless of your duty to the individual patient, the secondary public health consequences of losing general confidence (in, for example, communicable disease) are significant. Any disclosure therefore should be in the areas specified by the law and the patient should be made aware of these obligations when seeking treatment.

In the context of very specific legislation and professional guidance there would not appear much leeway for ethical debate, but circumstances regularly arise that do not fall unequivocally within such guidance. When the HIV-positive patient does not intend to inform his wife of his condition, or the unstable diabetic with recurrent hypoglycaemic seizures has not informed the DVLA, a delicate balance needs to be struck between maintaining patient confidence and avoiding broader harms. Although such decisions are taken at a senior medical level, confidentiality remains an active issue for all junior doctors; for example, limiting any transfer of medical information to that absolutely required by the treating team. We have a fundamental human weakness for sharing interesting knowledge from both a medical and a personal perspective, and whilst the first perspective may be considered integral to education and learning, even this sits within a very grey area of guidance.

ACTIVITY 11.2 A REAL STORY FROM AN ANAESTHETIC REGISTRAR

We have a daily trauma list printed with names, dates of birth, what operation is required etc. These are widely distributed to the wards, doctors, trauma coordinators and theatres. On numerous occasions I have found copies of the list on the corridor floor, obviously fallen out of busy person's pocket. I have only just started to realise the implications of this, that any passerby could pick it up and the breach in many patients confidentiality that could occur.

- Think about the last time you were in a lift at work. Did you or others discuss patient care?
- When you write in patients' notes or on a computer console looking up results, are you completely sure that no one else can see the information?

The next day you are at work, for just 30 minutes note how often patient confidentiality may have been, or was, breached. It can be an eye-opener!

Aspects of practice where doctors may find themselves inadvertently vulnerable to criticism include: not informing patients that personal information will be stored or passed on, sharing passwords for results servers or not logging off after accessing results, leaving medical records accessible to third parties or failing to ensure that discarded handover documentation has been rendered indecipherable by actions such as shredding. These scenarios highlight the very detailed and prescriptive guidance on the handling of patient data subsequent to the Data Protection Act of 1998. The Act contains eight 'Data Protection Principles' which specify that personal data must be:

- processed fairly and lawfully;

- obtained for specified and lawful purposes;

- adequate, relevant and not excessive;

- accurate and up to date;

- not kept any longer than necessary;

- processed in accordance with the 'data subject's' (the individual's) rights;

- securely kept;

- not transferred to any other country without adequate protection in situ.

> (see Information Commissioner's Office (ICO) for a guide to using the Data Protection Act and its principles, **www.ico.gov.uk/for_ organisations/data_protection/the_guide.aspx**)

Many doctors fail to realise that if they process personal data which could identify a living individual (where processing includes everything from acquisition to deletion of the data), they are in effect a data controller and should be registered with the Information Commissioner's Office (**www.ico.gov.uk**).

Secondary review of the core principles was undertaken by the Caldicott Committee in the light of increasing use of information technology systems. Any individual recording, storing or sharing of patient identifiable information should ensure compliance with the additional six principles.

i. Justify the purpose.
ii. Don't use patient identifiable information unless it is absolutely necessary.
iii. Use the minimum necessary patient identifiable information.
iv. Access to patient identifiable information should be on a strict need to know basis.
v. Everyone should be aware of their responsibilities.
vi. Understand and comply with the law.

> (Department of Health, 1997)

The inherent vulnerability of portable devices to loss or theft has led to further review and refinement; now all patient identifiable data stored on these devices must be encrypted. It is exceptionally easy when preparing or reviewing discharge letters, crafting a case report, presentation, information for a mortality meeting, or undertaking audit, to overlook these principles and inadvertently jeopardise professional credibility as well as compromising your primary ethical responsibility to the patient.

Case study 11.1: Mobile technologies and data protection

An elderly patient is admitted with a fractured neck of femur and unfortunately dies on day five without having an operation for a combination of factors including a weekend and other surgical priorities. You are asked to write a report for the coroner, the first occasion this has happened. Your consultant is on leave and has asked you to send a copy of the report to his home e-mail address before you send it to the coroner. You have started to write the report on a Trust computer but have not finished it and have saved it on the desktop and e-mailed a copy to your home address to complete the report at home. Your partner is a recently qualified lawyer and wants to make sure your report does not leave you vulnerable to criticism from the coroner or your employing Trust. You take the hospital notes home.

- Have you violated any law or professional guidelines related to confidentiality and if so how?
- Have you violated any laws related to data protection?
- If so, what are the potential penalties?
- What is the position of your consultant in relation to these issues?
- What sources of advice on these matters are there?

Conscientious objection

The law and professional guidelines on conscientious objection are quite clear, namely that no patient should be denied access to any form of treatment or assistance to which they are legitimately entitled, simply because of the individual beliefs of a healthcare practitioner (General Medical Council, 2008). This translates into a responsibility to ensure provision of care from a practitioner without such beliefs, or to provide the service directly. The subject has triggered intense debate on doctors' role, with some suggesting that a doctor's conscience has no place in a modern regulated healthcare system (Savulescu, 2006). Whilst an immediate consumer may support that view, it has to be considered that without a conscience, a doctor is simply an automaton of the state and is unlikely to be sensitively attuned to the additional ethical responsibilities of the profession which create obvious benefit for the patient, vocational fulfilment for the doctor, and therefore professional sustainability. The pragmatic middle ground is that it is crucial to informed debate with all relevant parties that doctors express their views on a range of sensitive issues such as termination of pregnancy, assisted conception and euthanasia. It is also important to ensure that decision-making by regulatory bodies and policy-makers follows an ethically defensible template when defining public policy. It remains unacceptable, however, for any doctor paid from public funds to make decisions which reflect their own particular beliefs rather than a patient's legitimate needs.

Conduct

Over the last five years, an interesting debate has been whether the conduct of medical students should be judged against the standard expected for doctors or that anticipated for the rest of the student population. It appears clear that where there is an interface with patients, or the profession is being represented, the same ethical standards as set out above pertain. Conduct also covers a range of other personal behaviours, some directly related to the patient interface, others related to the broader discharge of professional responsibilities, and others completely independent of your role as a doctor. For many of these areas, there is no comprehensive and unambiguous guidance, leaving the practitioner vulnerable to reactive criticism and significant sanctions if they have not considered the potential repercussions beforehand.

Cheating during examinations or falsification of information to gain an advantage during employment applications is always going to be interpreted, not only as bringing the profession into disrepute, but also as lacking insight into this interpretation to a degree that would question the right to registration.

A challenging discussion relates to 'spontaneous' and 'minor' criminality such as alcohol or drug-related offences as a student, and whether these issues should be subjected to self-regulation within the profession. What is not explicit is whether the sanctions for offences should rise with increasing progression as either a student or a doctor. Whilst this would appear reasonable at first visit, there is no rule of human behaviour that can expect errors of judgement to be eliminated by a certain age. Doctors should, however, reflect on choices they may have to make in their professional and private life (such as what they put on social networking sites) and consider those which may fall short of public expectation. The GMC sets out guidance for medical students and practising doctors on expectations around conduct (GMC, 2010a; GMC, 2006a).

Many of you will ultimately be responsible for an error, an avoidable complication of treatment or some other shortfall in care and have an accompanying responsibility to document this within the medical records and to inform the patient or their next of kin. Will you be able to discharge these responsibilities with integrity? In the event of an adverse outcome, will you be able to accept responsibility without allocation of blame to some other healthcare team member, or without some modification of the medical records which offers a more favourable interpretation of events?

Alongside these ongoing professional responsibilities, qualification poses additional challenges in the form of career progression particularly as we address for the first time a surplus of graduates over available foundation year posts. Embellishment of CVs and research fraud are obvious examples that cross a boundary, but at what stage does seeking insider information on selection process and marketing oneself to maximal effect become somehow unethical? Qualification also brings an introduction to unedifying behaviour within the profession, with many examples of violation of core ethical principles. As a newly qualified doctor, you will be placed in the difficult position of either silent complicity or professional isolation in the aftermath of whistle blowing. Practitioners may argue that these issues are simply those of personal integrity rather than of competing ethical principles, but you will need to consider how they will be addressed, whether this be receipt of hospitality from a pharmaceutical company, conflict of interest in relation to equipment purchases, abuse of charity or research funds, fraudulent expense claims, bullying within a clinical team, or persistent patient harms from direct incompetence or failure of process, such as ineffective handover procedure.

Case study 11.2: It is not as simple as first appears …

Regarding the above report for the coroner (Case study 11.1: Mobile technologies and data protection), your review of the medical records reveals that the patient's Warfarin, for her atrial fibrillation, was stopped on admission. She received no other form of DVT prophylaxis. You are not aware of the post-mortem findings. There has been no communication by medical staff with the next of kin. You e-mail your consultant with this information, asking for advice. He rings you back and instructs you to delete the e-mail, only communicate directly by telephone, and make no reference to these issues in the report, which is to be kept purely factual giving your grade and qualification, the patient's name and details, date of admission, presenting pathology and time and nature of death.

- What are your responsibilities in this situation to:
  - The next of kin?
  - The coroner?
  - Your consultant?
  - Your employer?

- What sources of advice have you access to?
- How do you resolve any conflict between your primary duties as a doctor and the accepted principle of following a consultant's instructions?
- What course of action do you take with regard to the coroner's report?

Ongoing ethical challenges

Ethical challenges that cannot simply be solved by reference to the law or professional guidelines will remain present within many clinical fields. Patients will continue to present to emergency medicine having taken an overdose and either refusing active intervention directly or being accompanied by an advance directive setting out the same position. Delayed resuscitation of cardiac arrest will continue to create a population with profound neurological injury. Neonatal intensive care teams will continue to rescue the extremely premature with the inevitability of severe and complex disability and the associated longer-term requirement for critical care blocking access to ICU beds for those who might benefit more from such care. Genetic advances will facilitate the treatment of inherited conditions and overcome infertility, but with inherent potential harms to both patient and wider population. Pandemic flu may become a reality, with the multiple problems of a depleted healthcare team, inadequate supplies, patient numbers in excess of available critical care resources, and challenging triage decisions being required.

These scenarios will create additional complex problems for the practitioner, when deciding on their own personal safety or the well-being of their family. Who has the authority to determine when and why a practitioner's responsibility to patients overrides that to their family in these circumstances?

Conflict

Differences of opinion will continue between healthcare providers and between providers and next of kin as to whether life-sustaining medical treatment should be initiated or continued. Some of these issues will be beyond internal resolution and appear before the courts, and it is appropriate to evaluate how the law approaches these matters, given the declared authority as set out at the beginning of this chapter.

For a problem to be addressed by the courts, an application has to be placed by one party or another, and ultimately the courts will decide whether the application can be considered lawful or otherwise. The court does not consider the rights or wrongs of the circumstances in which the application arose, does not offer mediation of differences of opinion between parties, and does not therefore resolve fundamental problems of understanding or communication that may underpin the dispute. It has been suggested therefore by media commentators that the courts are not the appropriate environment or process for addressing these life or death decisions (*The Times*, 2004). This demands a structure to anticipate, avoid and manage conflict, which goes beyond individual expertise and requires an institutional approach incorporating clinical ethics committees, an active patient advocacy service, genuinely independent second opinions, a forum for multidisciplinary discussion on problematical cases and consistency of medical approach.

Resolution of ethical problems by the courts

Attempts to reach a definitive legal solution for complex ethical problems often demonstrate shortcomings in legal process. When the withdrawal of nutrition and hydration from Anthony Bland, a Hillsborough victim, was declared lawful, such therapy had to be defined as artificial medical treatment rather than basic care, and the proposed course of action had to be interpreted as having the unwanted consequence of causing the patient's death, rather than this being the primary intention (*Airedale NHS Trust v Bland*, 1993). Perhaps the greatest shortcoming whilst euthanasia remains unlawful was the sanctioning of bringing about a patient's death by one of the most inhumane methods within a healthcare setting: starvation and dehydration. Whilst declaring this course of action lawful, paradoxically there was no generalisation on this point beyond the specific case but rather, an explicit expectation that any future similar cases should come before the court, and without this the strategy would remain unlawful. This judgement demonstrated an inherent lack of logic in that it is not within any court's power to declare lawful a course of action which is essentially unlawful.

Another example where the law struggled to be absolutely consistent was in the case of Ms B, a patient rendered quadriplegic and ventilator dependant via a tracheostomy, who wished artificial ventilation to be discontinued even though being aware of the inevitable consequence of death (*Ms B v an NHS Hospital Trust*, 2002). Despite the opposition of the treating medical team who argued that Ms B lacked capacity, the court was prepared to sanction this course of action and uphold the right to autonomy. At this point there is harmony between the law and ethical principles, but subsequent events in the form of transfer of the patient to an alternative hospital specifically for this purpose, the administration of sedative therapy prior to removal of ventilatory support, and the act of withdrawal, could be collectively interpreted as euthanasia or assisting a suicide, both of which remain unlawful in the UK. The deliberations of the court would have been very interesting therefore if medical opposition to the patient's wishes had been based on concerns as to lawfulness rather than the patient's capacity.

Case study 11.3: End-of-life care in complex situations

You are the F2 on the gastroenterology team caring for a 43-year-old patient previously diagnosed with advanced alcoholic liver disease. She presented with pneumonia three days ago which has progressed despite antibiotic therapy and is now complicated by encephalopathy, hypotension and oliguria. Your consultant has asked you to refer the patient to intensive care for all invasive support, emphasising her young age and teenage children. The consultant has already explained this course of action to the patient's husband. The intensive care registrar reviews the patient and states that there is no available bed and that in any case he would not be admitting her because of the poor prognosis and futility.

- Who has authority for decision-making in these circumstances?
- What is the role of the next of kin in this situation?
- Who should make a decision regarding the appropriateness of intensive care provision, the parent specialty or intensive care practitioners?
- What sources of advice are available?
- Is the nature of the patient's underlying condition of alcohol dependence relevant when making decisions about the utilisation of scarce resources?
- What options are available to the next of kin if they do not agree with the intensive care position?

- Would the intensive care team be under any duty to initiate life-sustaining medical treatment pending an application by the family to the courts?
- What factors would be incorporated into a 'best interests' decision and what weighting should be given to these different factors?

Conclusions

Medical ethics can be interpreted in a variety of ways from an academic growth industry to providing essential guidance in the light of medical advances and changing societal expectations. For the everyday clinician, the law and professional guidance remains the appropriate point of reference, but every aspect of our interface with patients and colleagues, and our own personal conduct should go beyond simply considering what is expected by law and be based on maximising patient and public trust and confidence.

An understanding of the basic principles of medical ethics can help with discussion and decision-making, but perhaps the greatest benefit is to recognise when we are in an 'ethical' dilemma and use our understanding to behave with consistent professional integrity.

Chapter summary

- Ethical issues and dilemmas form part of everyday clinical practice.

- An understanding of the relationship between ethics, the law, personal beliefs and professional guidance will help you become a more effective and mindful doctor.

- A range of resources will help support you in dealing with ethical issues.

GOING FURTHER

Beauchamp, TL and Childress, JF (2001) *Principles of Biomedical Ethics,* 5th edition. Oxford: Oxford University Press.
A comprehensive text which addresses issues of morality, medical ethics, informed consent and other ethical areas.

Danbury, C, Newdick, C, Waldmann, C and Lawson, A (eds) (2010) *Law and Ethics in Intensive Care*. Oxford: Oxford University Press.
This book gives an up-to-date outline of how the law has changed and how this has affected the practice of intensive care medicine. Clinical scenarios illustrate actual problems that arise during normal clinical practice.

chapter 12

The Legal Framework of Medical Practice
Dominic Bell

Achieving foundation competences

This chapter will help you begin to meet the following requirements of the *Foundation Programme Curriculum* (2010)

Competences

F1

- Discusses the risks of legal and disciplinary action if a doctor fails to achieve the necessary standards of practice and care.
- Describes and applies the principles of:
  - confidentiality;
  - child protection procedures;
  - completes death certificates and liaises with the coroner/procurator fiscal;
  - completes cremation forms appropriately;
  - minimises risk of exposing a pregnant woman to radiation;
  - recognises the need for restraint of some patients with mental illness according to the appropriate legal framework.

F2

- Discusses the implications of a living will or advance directive.
- Initiates restraining orders in some patients with mental illness according to the appropriate legal framework.

Knowledge

- Legal framework that relates to medical practice and its application to patient management.
- The Mental Health Act (1983) section 5 (2) and Mental Health Care and Treatment (2003) Scotland.
- The Mental Capacity Act (2005) England and Wales. Adults with Incapacity Act (2000) Scotland.
- The Data Protection Act 1998 and Freedom of Information Act 2002 in Scotland and 2005 in England as well as UK and European legislation relating to access to records.
- Legal responsibilities for completing death certificates.

- Types of death to be referred to the coroner/procurator fiscal.
- The doctor's role in cremation procedures.
- Situations where compulsory detention under a section of mental health legislation in the UK would be appropriate.
- Conditions that patients should report to the DVLA, and doctors' responsibilities if they fail to do so.
- The role of medical evidence in the coroner's court and other legal proceedings.
- Basic knowledge of equalities legislation and its impact on medical practice linked to equality duty in regard to race, disability and gender.
- Child protection procedures, inter-agency referral routes (e.g. police, social services) and when to involve them.
- Legal framework surrounding justification of exposure to ionising radiation by referring practitioner.

Chapter overview

The amount of knowledge about medical law that is required at first appears enormous. With so many laws, acts and principles it can be overwhelming. However, many (not all) pertain to how you would behave in real life as a professional person whereas other legal rules help with complicated medical situations. This chapter cannot contain all the information required from the competencies above but discusses where the law supports professional practice and when conflicts arise between the professions.

After reading this chapter you will be able to:

- describe the key features of medical law as they apply to practice;
- apply the law in practical situations with key client groups;
- identify situations when legal rules, ethics and professional guidance comes into conflict;
- identify areas of law that you need to learn more about and know where to obtain guidance.

Introduction

Medical students and doctors can acquire a jaundiced view of lawyers, stereotyping their predatory opportunism and greed, but fearing their power to destroy a doctor's reputation in the courtroom. The very concept of law is also often interpreted negatively as an intrusive threat to the medical profession by emphasising doctors' duties and patients' rights (Preston-Shoot and McKimm, 2010). Many factors prevent rationalisation of these views, not least of which is that medical law has to compete with a host of other responsibilities for a clinician's attention, as this book emphasises. A recent study suggests that medical students' overall perception of the law is positive. A sound understanding of law is seen as essential, enabling doctors to achieve health improvements, protect vulnerable people and demonstrate accountability. However, concerns persist about defensive practice, keeping updated, the synergy between law and medical values, and applying legal rules (Preston-Shoot et al., 2011).

The goal of this chapter is to set out some of the rules that not only govern but also help to guide our practice, understand the driving principles behind these, and hopefully stimulate engagement with a field that offers greater opportunity than threat. The 'Going further' section provides examples of where you can go to extend your knowledge and understanding of the law.

ACTIVITY 12.1 YOUR THOUGHTS ON MEDICAL LAW

- What has been your previous interaction with medical law?
- How would you describe your view of 'the law'?
- Do you dread the time you may get called to coroner's court?

The law as applicable to medicine

Traditional views assumed an imbalance in the relationship between doctor and patient. Whilst this is changing, for many the doctor is portrayed as knowledgeable, powerful and prone to paternalism, whilst the patient is perceived as vulnerable, not only by the presenting illness and its impact on employment, relationships and responsibilities, but also by relative ignorance induced by social divide. Education on ethical principles should ensure that these issues are understood and addressed, and the General Medical Council as regulatory body specifies the duties of a doctor in this area which are mandated as a condition of registration.

The law similarly takes the position that a patient needs to be protected and dictates that a patient should have access to all available therapies, participate in fully informed consent, and have rights of redress if the standard of care falls below an acceptable level. Whilst not specifying the attitudes expected of you, the law clearly prohibits any discrimination based on race, gender, disability or sexual orientation. Aspects of the professional relationship other than direct clinical care are also regulated, covering confidentiality and research, and there are numerous responsibilities after death covering certification of death, retention of tissue and other biological material, post-mortem examinations and organ donation.

These multiple duties come under particular scrutiny when dealing with the most vulnerable members of society such as adults lacking capacity and individuals with no next of kin, and recent statute in the form of the Mental Capacity Act carries the sanction of custodial sentence for breaches. The management of patients with a mental health disorder is tightly regulated under the Mental Health Act 2007, which specifies when restraint and compulsory institutionalisation can be deployed and which conditions can be treated against the patient's will.

Children are another vulnerable group and the Children Act 1989 specifies the obligation on any organisation or individual to prevent harm, translating in turn to be aware of the potential for harm, consider the possibility in any interface and follow the appropriate course of action in the event of concerns. Regulation also covers diverse and often overlooked populations other than the above main groups with for example obligations to avoid ionising radiation during pregnancy as set out by the Health Protection Agency (in its standards (Health Protection Agency (HPA) Standards, **www.hpa.org.uk**).

Certain specific responsibilities after death such as certification, liaison with the coroner and completion of cremation forms, are also regulated by the law and currently subjected to critical scrutiny following the malevolent actions of Shipman and other healthcare workers. The law also oversees the regulation of doctors, with recent tightening of procedure following evidence of significant shortfalls in the GMC's handling of Shipman's registration. As a doctor, you are also bound by 'common law' which covers, for example, prohibition of euthanasia as well as more 'mundane' criminal activity such as assault, theft or fraud. Whilst you may reasonably consider an interface with the law in any of the above circumstances a stressful and sometimes hostile occurrence, many clinicians routinely interact with judicial process without there being a presumption of practitioner guilt, such as mental health tribunals, the coroner's court or the Court of Protection.

The law and direct clinical care

The key issues in this field are access to treatment, consent and standards of care.

Access to treatment

Despite the Human Rights Act, the law does not grant every patient access to every form of treatment, there being recognition that funding authorities have to prioritise to maximise overall health gain for the population they serve and that certain treatments may be restricted on health economic grounds by agencies such as NICE (**www.nice.org.uk**). Any decision has, however, to be compliant with European law in which discrimination is prohibited, thereby preventing any restriction on care due to age, religion or sexual orientation, a concept which has led (for example) to successful appeals for assisted conception by lesbian couples. The flip-side of such evaluations is that in avoiding discrimination against certain patient groups and setting objective physiological or pathological parameters as a trigger for an intervention, patients may be inadvertently denied more appropriate treatment. This is illustrated by patients 'choosing' to increase their BMI to greater than 50 to meet the threshold for bariatric surgery, rather than complying with lifestyle advice on dietary restriction and exercise.

These issues can place you in a difficult position when deciding how to maximise the efficacy and efficiency of available resources, and in exercising professional judgement as to what is in the best interests of the patient. Should certain treatment options not be discussed if they are not reasonably accessible and should care be reduced to referring for a specific treatment simply because this is a 'legal right' within national guidelines? Once the legal position is understood, and there is compliance with guidelines from the GMC, these aspects assume an ethical dimension, see Chapter 11.

Consent

The concept of consent, as a dynamic process is founded in an individual's right to autonomy. Consent remains orientated towards interventionist and surgical procedures as opposed to other types of investigations such as lumbar puncture, central venous access, and blood transfusions. These other types of procedures can have just as serious complications and implications as surgical procedures but are often not approached in a similar manner.

The position at law is that any intervention which carries a risk or which constitutes an invasion of privacy would meet the legal criteria for requiring consent. This involves an explanation of what is proposed and why, which includes the relative risks and benefits of alternative approaches, including doing nothing. When determining which risks are to be relayed to the patient, the legal expectation after the case of *Chester v Afshar* (2004) is not what the doctor believes to be significant either numerically or in terms of impact, but what the patient would consider significant. This translates into your obligation to provide written and where appropriate pictorial information on the nature and frequency of the known risks, an interval for the patient to consider those risks, and an opportunity to further discuss the risks the patient considers relevant, all in the light of the practitioner's own experience and expertise.

ACTIVITY 12.2 WHO IS THE BEST PERSON TO OBTAIN CONSENT?

For the following three scenarios think about whether you would be happy to take the consent and what issues you would have to consider in making that decision.

You are asked to go see a patient and take consent for:

- a gastroscopy;
- a total hip replacement;
- an aortic valve replacement.

There are many routine procedures where you may be happy to obtain consent provided the patient has capacity. However, you should know the limits of your own competence in obtaining consent and seek advice and training if needed. One answer to who is the best person to obtain consent is that it depends on the procedure, but it also might depend on the patients' capacity, their previous history or experiences and their culture.

The current position in healthcare litigation is that even if a known complication materialises and there is no evidence that the treatment or intervention was negligently conducted, the patient would have a valid claim for compensation if there was no documentary evidence to confirm that the process had been diligently followed.

Standards of care: negligence

The law also exists to protect patients from the harms of medical interventions if these meet the criteria for negligence, and redress may take the form of financial compensation and, more rarely, criminal proceedings if the outcome has been fatal. A successful claim requires proof that there was a breach in the duty of care which was owed to the patient, and the likelihood on a balance of probability, which may be as little as 51–49, that the adverse outcome arose from that breach. It is interesting, however, that if the negligence caused death or injury which was still more likely than not to occur regardless of the negligent act, there is no redress for such a 'loss of opportunity' (*Hotson* v *East Berkshire Area Health Authority*, 1987). This interpretation is often active in cases involving delayed diagnosis of malignancy. Certain additional principles have been derived through case law which do benefit the claimant, whereby inexperience on the part of a practitioner or a lack of facilities on the part of an institution are not a defence, since provision of services should be based on the predictable needs of the patient population that is served (*Wilsher* v *Essex Area Health Authority*, 1988).

These principles are not absolute however, and the drivers behind increasing sub-specialisation, namely to improve the standard of care on a routine basis, may prevent such care being available out of hours or during annual leave. It is increasingly common for cases such as ruptured aortic aneurysm that would have been previously operated on by the on-call general surgeon to be transferred out of a district hospital to a regional centre. Such changes in service delivery might lead to a death during transfer which might be an undesirable but inevitable and probably defensible consequence.

An additional difficulty in defining an adverse outcome as negligent arises from the lack of any specialty standards which specifically identify when certain outcomes, in certain categories of patient, reflect a shortfall in competence or performance which would meet the criteria for negligence.

To be successful, a claimant has to prove such a breach of duty using the Bolam threshold whereby, 'A doctor is not guilty of negligence if he has acted in accordance with a practice accepted as proper by a responsible body of medical men skilled in that particular art ... Putting it the other way around, a doctor is not negligent if he is acting in accordance with such a practice, merely because there is a body of opinion that takes the contrary view' (*Bolam* v *Friern Hospital Management Committee*, 1957). It has been argued that this is not an unequivocal template which can be applied, but a matter of opinion, and the majority of claims have failed historically when a senior and usually academic doctor states for the defence: 'it is not how I would have provided treatment, but that does not define the care as going beyond that expected of a reasonably competent practitioner'. This demonstrates the randomness of civil procedure, and explains the number of unsuccessful claims and the frustration of a worthy claimant thwarted by the court craft of experienced defence experts.

The inherent inconsistencies, protracted timescale and exceptional cost through legal fees to the public purse have resulted in reforms to civil procedure, setting out rules on disclosure, time limits for completion of key stages, and allowing for the joint instruction of a single expert. Whilst some progress has been made, the adversarial nature of these proceedings remains, if only because doctors do not wish to concede that their practice has been negligent, they have access to professional indemnity with defence societies usually able to access a supportive opinion, and because the onus falls on the claimant to prove negligence.

The last decade has, however, seen a partial move away from *Bolam* with gradual adoption of the *Bolitho* (*Bolitho* v *City and Hackney Health Authority*, 1997) principle, whereby clinical practice is expected to be refined over time by the adoption of strategies that maximise the likelihood of success and minimise the risk of complications. A relevant example for junior doctors would be the use of ultrasound guidance for central line insertion, as endorsed by the National Institute for Clinical Excellence (NICE, 2002) wherein if a patient suffered complications of carotid puncture whilst using a landmark-based technique, this is now unlikely to be defensible unless the line was sited in an absolute emergency with no immediate access to a functional ultrasound machine. *Bolitho* also established the principle that expert opinion had to be logical and to accommodate advances in medical practice, such that the traditional *Bolam* defence as set out above would be under scrutiny and leave the expert vulnerable to judicial censure.

The reality is, however, that the status quo, which largely favours the defendant, has essentially been maintained and attempts to introduce alternative systems, such as no-fault compensation, have been severely restricted. At this point in time therefore, no party except lawyers are served well by an industry which is persistently grounded in an adversarial approach, a power imbalance between experts, and individual interpretation and opinion rather than objective and explicit criteria against which to judge an adverse outcome.

Standards of care: gross negligence manslaughter

If a patient death arises from medical error or some shortfall in care, particularly if the incident has been the subject of national warnings or defined by the National Patient Safety Agency as a 'never event' such as wrong site surgery, the default position of many coroners is to request a police investigation into 'gross negligence manslaughter'. The criterion used for this assessment is whether; 'the negligence of the accused went beyond a mere matter of compensation between subjects and showed such disregard for the life and safety of others as to amount to a crime against the state and conduct deserving punishment' (*R* v *Bateman*, 1925).

The majority of successful prosecutions in the UK have involved junior doctors from overseas, and when all the circumstances of a case are examined, questions can be asked over the orientation and induction programmes, assessment of competence, specification of responsibilities, explicit and unambiguous protocols for care, and senior supervision of these individuals, which cumulatively would constitute serious system failures rather than sole individual culpability. The greatest societal harm is caused by scapegoating an individual rather than addressing the more fundamental causes.

The opportunity to target system failures and organisational flaws is now possible under the Corporate Manslaughter and Corporate Homicide Act 2007, but given the potential penalties for senior managers, it is likely that the defence strategy will be to devolve responsibility to individual staff members. This strategy has been apparent in previous prosecution of hospitals by the Health and Safety Executive (HSE) under the Health and Safety at Work Act, emphasising the importance of junior doctors having independent professional indemnity rather than relying on cover provided by the employer (*R* v *Southampton University Hospital Trust*, 2006).

Broader professional responsibilities

Confidentiality

Although the duty of confidentiality is addressed in Chapter 11 on ethical aspects of practice, it must be emphasised that doctors are governed very specifically by the law on this issue. Patients come to you for advice and treatment at vulnerable stages in their lives, and the law stipulates confidentiality unless the information is specifically required to be disclosed. Such scenarios include reporting of transmissible disease or adverse drug reactions, liaison with the DVLA on conditions such as epilepsy if an individual continues to drive against medical advice (**www.dft.gov.uk/dvla**) and certain injuries to children that warrant engagement of the protection agencies. Additionally, if a patient presents with gunshot or knife wounds, the police should be informed as soon as feasible since they have responsibility for ensuring the ongoing safety of the patient and to limit the risk to other members of the community, including the healthcare team providing treatment (General Medical Council, 2009b).

The duty of confidentiality has received additional attention recently in the light of practitioners accessing the electronic radiological images, investigations and records of individuals with a high public profile, a process capable of triggering a range of sanctions including criminal charges, a civil claim, disciplinary action by the employer and scrutiny by the regulatory bodies. You need therefore to be aware of your responsibilities under the Data Protection Act and the Medical Records Act, and the importance of not carrying any patient identifiable data on any portable device unless absolutely essential and encrypted.

Respect for the human body

The Alder Hey retained organs scandal demonstrated how the medical profession had persistently failed to understand and accommodate the public's perception on how the dead should be treated. This shortcoming was radically addressed within new legislation, the Human Tissue Act (HT Act), wherein the retention of even a microscope slide of tissue had to be justified and the subject of fully informed consent. The restrictive impact of this approach on future research was recognised as the bill went through parliament with some concessions made, but all practitioners will face the more common consequence of the Act when requesting post-mortem examinations. A similar standard of consent is expected to that set out above for operative procedures, with provision of written information, the opportunity to ask questions or reconsider the decision, liaison with the pathologist as to the undertakings, and comprehensive documentation of process.

Organ donation

Doctors may consider that the concept of organ donation, particularly if it involves tissue harvesting of skin and bone, raises interesting questions in relation to the above principles, primarily because the same standard of consent for a post-mortem is rarely approached for donation. There is paradoxical authorisation under the HT Act to automatically consider any patient who has been certified dead as a potential organ donor and interventions deemed lawful without any requirement for the consent of the next of kin include aortic and venous cannulation to deliver cold perfusion of the splanchnic organs prior to retrieval. The profession is entering an era where the needs of recipients and the viability of the transplantation industry create challenges to our primary responsibility to the patient and to maintaining public confidence that our goal will remain their survival (Bell, 2010b). Conversion rates from death to donation are being scrutinised, Trusts are being evaluated on this basis, organ donation champions have been appointed with the role of maximising recruitment and trained facilitators are employed to increase consent rates from the next of kin. With recent declarations that it is lawful to undertake certain interventions on patients prior to death to optimise the chances of successful transplantation after death (Department of Health, 2009), it can be seen that this activity will continue to present interesting challenges for clinicians as they seek to support government initiatives without jeopardising public confidence or their own reputations.

Case study 12.1: Consent and capacity

Mina, an 89-year-old woman with dementia and agitated depression attended the gastro clinic because of bleeding PR which had been noted by her carers. In the last two months she has lost two stone in weight and had a large abdominal mass. The specialist registrar (SpR) did not feel that further investigation or treatment would affect the outcome in this case, but after talking with her son over the telephone, decided to admit her for a gastric endoscopy and colonoscopy. As you arrive on the ward, you hear Mina shouting out that she wants to go home. A message has been left that 'the son will consent for the procedures'. How do you proceed?

This case study raises issues around how doctors and other health professionals obtain consent from vulnerable people. The next section explores this further.

Vulnerable members of society

Loss of capacity

It is important that doctors respect individual patient choice but this leaves patients lacking competence for decision-making in an extremely vulnerable position. The state historically recognised this vulnerability and the monarch assumed the role of 'parens patriae' or 'parent of the nation' until this was inadvertently lost under the Mental Health Act 1959. This legislation left no one, including the courts and the next of kin, able to consent to medical treatment on behalf of an incompetent patient, except for a mental health disorder. The principles of 'necessity' and 'best interests' which guide treatment for these individuals were subsequently derived through case law, and after a protracted evolution, the Mental Capacity Act (MCA) finally received royal assent in 2005 (Bell, 2007). The key components relate to the assessment of capacity, assistance towards autonomous decision-making where possible, and the processes to be followed once lack of capacity is confirmed.

Case study 12.2: Consent and capacity continued

You go to assess Mina prior to her procedures and find that she is agitated and that it is impossible to have a conversation with her. The only thing you can determine is that she does not believe you are a doctor and this is not the hospital. It is obvious to you that Mina does not have the capacity to give or withhold consent, since she appears unable at this moment to understand, retain, believe and weigh the relevant information, even in a limited form.

- How would you proceed?
- Who would you need to contact?

If a patient lacking capacity has no identifiable next of kin, an independent mental capacity advocate (IMCA) must be instructed and if decisions have to be made over a sustained period of time, the Court of Protection will appoint a deputy to oversee the process of care.

Planning for loss of capacity

Under the Mental Capacity Act, individuals are able to plan ahead for the time they may lack capacity with either advance directives or through empowering an individual with lasting power of attorney (LPA) with authority for personal welfare. For an advance directive to be binding it must be in writing, signed, dated and witnessed at a time when the patient had capacity, must be applicable to the clinical scenario facing the clinician, and must be comprehensive and unambiguous in the declarations. Specific cases illustrate the difficulties and subsequent criticisms when doctors either adhere to the instructions (BMJ Group blogs, 2009), or deviate from them (Bonner et al., 2009). Although the principle of self-determination should be paramount, a unilateral declaration potentially many years before the clinical events may fail to accommodate advances in medical care or a change in the patient's position. There is evidence that given this option the public elect not to generate a fixed and binding directive but prefer flexible decision-making by healthcare team and next of kin in the light of all available evidence at that current time (Perkins, 2007).

A lasting power of attorney is theoretically authoritative under the MCA even with regards to life-sustaining medical treatment (LSMT), if this particular aspect is specified, but practitioners should note that any position adopted by an LPA either to continue or withhold LSMT can be challenged if it is not considered to be in the best interests of the patient by the healthcare team.

Restraint and restrictions

The MCA has a strong focus on avoiding any restriction on a patient whether through physical or chemical restraint, retaining a patient within an institution through measures such as locked doors, or a form of treatment which may restrict future choice, such as sterilisation. Any restriction should therefore be absolutely essential to protect the patient from harm, must be proportional to that potential harm, should be reviewed on a regular basis and stopped or modified as the risk reduces. However, the MCA does not prohibit physical restraint, and there is an understanding that at times this may be essential for the protection of the team rather than the patient and because logistically it is impossible to provide continuous surveillance of and attendance on an individual patient.

Duties and penalties

It is not feasible to set out a solution for every potential scenario, and the debate on advance directives shows how aspects of the new legislation remain open to different interpretations. Although the MCA comes with the authority of a custodial sentence for non-compliance, it is anticipated that this would only be applicable for deviation from the primary principles, rather than flaws in the decision reached. On this basis, practitioners must demonstrate that they have made an assessment of capacity, sought multi-disciplinary consensus and second opinion, liaised with next of kin as to best interests, and comprehensively documented the process.

Mental health

Despite potential overlap, management of the patient with a mental health disorder is distinct from that of the individual lacking capacity, and set out in the Mental

Health Act 2007, which in essence is a series of amendments to the 1983 Act. Although an expanded range of healthcare professionals now have authority for the treatment of patients without their consent, it still requires specific training and licensing to section a patient and a series of safeguards exist, including mental health advocates and tribunals, which prevent indefinite detention. Furthermore, a patient cannot be detained unless they have a condition which has a recognised treatment, a specification which prevents the involuntary commitment of individuals with an antisocial personality disorder. It should also be noted that the presence of a mental health disorder does not inherently compromise capacity for other healthcare decisions and this creates a recurring problem for emergency departments when patients refuse treatment for an overdose or other variants of self-harm. The usual default position is to sedate the patient and expedite active treatment, but cases such as that of *Wooltorton* above, where the patient is in possession of an advance directive refusing such care, generate caution before this course of action.

Child protection

Every individual or agency with an interface with children has a responsibility to promote children's well-being, which for a doctor primarily translates into considering the possibility of neglect or abuse in its various forms regardless of the presenting condition. Each Trust has a designated child protection officer and it is likely that the subject will be a designated learning module as a condition of employment. The GMC as regulatory body specifies compliance with the principles of the Children Act as a condition of registration in *Good Medical Practice* and other professional bodies have contributed educational material such as *Child Protection: A tool kit for doctors* from the BMA (BMA, 2009b)

Disability

Another patient cohort identified as vulnerable are those with disability, particularly if the ability to communicate is compromised as in cerebral palsy. Protection for these individuals, particularly from discrimination, lies within the Human Rights Act, and doctors face a significant challenge when their concerns that treatment may simply prolong a life characterised by suffering, is interpreted as a paternalistic view on quality of life by next of kin. Avoiding recrimination and court involvement in these circumstances requires empathy, patience and the highest level of communication.

Research

International outrage at experimentation on human subjects in Nazi Germany triggered the Nuremberg Code and later refinement with the Declaration of Helsinki in 1974. Disclosures on American syphilis studies in Tuskegee and Guatemala (Fox, 2010) demonstrates how violation of these principles was not limited to extreme regimes and is the driver behind fully informed consent before research can be conducted or published. The interplay between research and the commercial world is another area coming under increasing scrutiny, with evidence of fraud and suppression of evidence relating to complications or lack of efficacy. Fraud is clearly a criminal matter but the responsibility of a doctor to inform the medical community of negative results which would otherwise go unpublished has to be balanced against the possibility of an expensive libel action by the relevant company (Henderson, 2009). Given additional rules on authorship and the interest of the General Medical Council as highlighted by erasure from the register in cases relating to the MMR vaccine (General Medical Council, 2010f), it is clear that research is a fraught area, but with career progression intertwined with publication, the associated pressure may well continue to generate flawed material and attract unfavourable attention.

End-of-life care

This vast area encompasses law, ethics and personal religious and secular beliefs which cannot be accommodated within this chapter. Junior doctors should, however, be aware of the core principles as defined by national law (Bell, 2007) and the recent directives from the GMC (Bell, 2010a), which collectively govern best practice.

ACTIVITY 12.3 END OF LIFE ASSISTANCE (SCOTLAND) BILL

Please read the following document:

www.scottish.parliament.uk/s3/bills/38-EndLifeAssist/b38s3-introd.pdf

The bill stipulates that terminally ill people who find life intolerable or those who are so permanently physically incapacitated that they cannot live independently and find life intolerable should be able to seek help from a doctor to end their lives.

• What do you think about this?

Where do you think your views have come from (for example, knowledge of the law, cultural or religious beliefs, your own moral code or professional guidance)?

In deciding what you think and how you might act, what other considerations might need to be taken in to account?

Clearly, issues relating to end-of-life care and euthanasia are very difficult to deal with, for patients, families and for the health professionals who care for them. Doctors, especially those working in different countries with different legal frameworks, will need to have clearly thought through their position on such legal and ethical situations so they can practice safely, yet with respect for patient's wishes.

Diverse responsibilities: certification of death and liaison with the coroner

Historically, confirmation and the subsequent certification of death was the responsibility of the most junior doctor available. This practice was exposed in the aftermath of Shipman and other healthcare workers who murdered patients (Leeds Teaching Hospitals NHS Trust, 2002), and trusts should have systems in place whereby all deaths are reviewed by a senior clinician before certification, request for a post-mortem or liaison with the coroner. If there is clear evidence from the history, clinical assessment and investigations that death was attributable to natural causes, and the patient has been in hospital for more than 24 hours, a medical certificate as to cause of death (MCCD) should be issued to allow funeral arrangements to proceed. The doctor is not expected to know the exact cause but to certify what is believed to be the cause. There is a pressure to complete the certificate, given public aversion to post-mortem examination, and an increasing shortage of pathologists undertaking routine hospital post-mortems.

Within the formal death certificate documentation, there is a comprehensive list of circumstances in which the death should be referred to the coroner, including complications of medical intervention regardless of whether these reflected any shortfall in care. A lesser-known obligation arises in the context of natural causes but where there was a lost opportunity to overt the outcome which should in normal circumstances have been taken. Case law dictates that such a death can be redefined as 'unnatural causes' and should be referred to the coroner (*R* v *Inner North London Coroner ex p Touche*, 2001). If the next of kin have expressed any reservations as to the standard of treatment, the question arises as to whether the death arose due to 'a lack of medical care', and it would also be wise to report such a death.

The completion of a form for cremation requires a high level of detail post-Shipman and practitioners can expect rigorous cross-examination from doctors signing Part 2 of the form or the crematorium referee.

It is interesting that there is no statutory definition of death within the UK, an observation highlighted by organ donation recruitment strategies which target the recently dead. The Academy of Medical Royal Colleges has recently produced guidance on this issue and when confirming death doctors should document the features specified and the timing of these observations (Academy of Medical Royal Medical Colleges, 2008).

The doctor and common law

Despite the abundance of statute governing the profession's interface with patients, doctors are more likely to fall foul of the law by engaging in basic criminal activity such as fraudulent expense claims, theft, perjury whilst giving evidence, assault, drug offences, or driving under the influence. Any criminal activity will automatically be referred to the GMC and can threaten freedom as well as livelihood and reputation.

The doctor and the courts

The above sections have emphasised how the law sets out rules for every dimension of our clinical practice and in view of potential sanctions it would be reasonable to view any court appearance as a threat. Not all courts are adversarial however: the coroner's court being inquisitorial and directed towards the determination of who the deceased was and where, when, and how they came by their death, with strict rules preventing self-incrimination or verdicts implying criminality or civil liability. The family courts are similarly directed towards the best interests of patients rather than challenging the actions and intentions of doctors, and whilst certain areas such as child protection are highly charged, the judgements in the majority of cases involving adults lacking capacity are based on consensus and mediation between all interested parties.

Overview and opportunities

These considerations emphasise the opportunity inherent in medical law for practitioners, whether as expert witnesses, coroners, defence society advisers, or even with additional training as solicitors or barristers. Many universities have established distant-learning programmes with masters' degrees in medical law and/or ethics. The Royal College of Physicians has recognised the potential for diversification within the profession and established the Faculty of Forensic and Legal Medicine with the mission to establish and maintain the highest standards of competence and integrity in this challenging field.

Doctors do need an understanding of the law not only in the light of your primary responsibility to patients, but also for your own protection and the reputation of the profession. The law does not, however, need to be viewed as a nebulous threat and should be interpreted as a series of helpful signposts that protect doctors and even an opportunity to expand your portfolio beyond clinical care.

Case study 12.3: Consent, capacity and testing

An F1 doctor who suspects she may be in the early stages of pregnancy sustains a needlestick injury whilst attempting cannulation of a combative and non-compliant patient who has sustained head and general injuries in an assault. There is clinical evidence that the patient is an intravenous drug abuser and this history has been recorded during previous emergency department admissions. There is no record of the patient's HIV or hepatitis status and no obvious indication to conduct these tests for the patient's benefit at this stage of the care pathway. Due to the presence of cerebral contusions on CT scan, treatment will require sedation for at least 48 hours and it is questionable whether the patient will ever regain full capacity for medical decision-making. It is obviously in the doctor's best interests to know the patient's virological status to make an informed choice about prophylaxis treatment which does carry certain risks.

- Which laws are active in relation to whether testing of the patient is permissible?
- Does any individual have the authority to test the patient without consent?
- Does any individual or body have the authority to consent or assent to testing on behalf of the patient?
- How (if at all) does the potential pregnancy of the doctor influence decision-making in this case?
- If testing was conducted, how would the law on confidentiality be adhered to in relation to communication and documentation of the result?
- What is the position of the GMC, BMA and defence societies on this subject?
- What are the possible consequences for any doctor who tests the patient for the benefit of the F1 doctor?
- What is the appropriate course of action for a doctor who is aware that testing has been conducted and believes this course of action to be unlawful?
- What are the potential adverse consequences for the patient, healthcare practitioners and society if testing is not permissible?
- What potential solutions are available in the context of the current laws and Department of Health initiatives in relation to organ donation, see **www.dh.gov.uk/en/Publicationsandstatistics/ Publications/PublicationsPolicyAndGuidance/DH_108825**.

Chapter summary

- An understanding of the law in relation to ethical and professional principles will give you a sound foundation for clinical practice.

- Key legal issues relating to the role of the doctor include consent, confidentiality, capacity, access to treatment, end of life care, certifying death and research.

- There are many places to go for help, find out locally where you can find out information and make yourself familiar with online resources.

- The law is constantly being reviewed and updated in response to social change and expectations, it is important to keep up to date with the law as it relates to medical practice.

GOING FURTHER

www.ethox.org.uk – very useful website with lots of reading and teaching material available to all.

Kennedy, I and Grubb, A (2000) *Medical Law,* 3rd edition. London: Butterworths.

Mason, K and Laurie, G (2011) *Mason and McCall Smith's Law and Medical Ethics,* 8th edition. New York: Oxford University Press.

part 4
Working Collaboratively

chapter 13

Collaboration and Interprofessional Working

Jill Thistlethwaite

Achieving foundation competences

This chapter will help you to begin to meet the following requirements of the *Foundation Programme Curriculum* (2010).

1.1 Behaviour in the workplace

Competences

- Always recognises own level of competence and asks for help from appropriate sources.
- Is courteous, polite and professional when communicating with both patients and colleagues.
- Encourages an atmosphere of open communication and appropriately directed communication within teams.
- Only shares clinical information, whether spoken or written, with appropriate individuals or groups.
- Seeks out role models and tries to learn from the behaviours of the best clinical practitioners and leaders.

1.3 Time management and continuity of care

Competences

F1

- Is punctual for start of shifts, meetings, handovers and other duties.
- Delegates or calls for help in a timely fashion when s/he is falling behind.
- Ensures satisfactory completion of tasks at the end of the shift/day with appropriate handover.

F2

- Demonstrates an ability to adjust decision-making in situations where staffing levels and support are reduced (e.g. out of hours).
- Is aware of work pressures on others and takes appropriate action to help reorganise workloads.

Knowledge

- Which patients/tasks take priority.
- Which patients/tasks need formal hand-over.
- Relevance of continuity of care.
- Personal and collective responsibility for patient welfare.

3.10 Ensures safe continuing care of patients on handover between shifts, on-call staff or with 'hospital at night' team by meticulous attention to detail and reflection on performance

Competences

F1

- Accurately summarises and documents the main points of patients' diagnoses, active problems, and management plans.
- Provides clear information to colleagues.
- Attends handovers punctually and accepts directions and allocation of tasks from seniors.

F2

- Supports colleagues in forward planning at handover.
- Can, and sometimes does, organise handover, briefing and task allocation.
- Anticipates potential problems for next shift and takes pre-emptive action.

7.3 Promotes patient safety through good team-working

Competences

F1 and F2

- Works in partnership with patients and colleagues to develop sustainable care plans to manage patients' acute and chronic conditions.
- Cross-checks instructions and actions with colleagues, e.g. medicines to be injected.
- Draws attention to risks or potential risks to patients regardless of status of colleagues.
- Describes ways of identifying and dealing with poor performance in self and colleagues, including senior colleagues.

14.2 Interface with different specialties and with other professionals

Competences

F1

- Shows an understanding of the challenges of providing optimum care within a variety of clinical settings.
- Arranges appropriate urgent investigations and chases results when necessary.

F2

- Consistently seeks effective communication with colleagues in other disciplines.
- Describes the process of referral from primary to secondary care.

Knowledge

- Effective team working.
- Roles and responsibilities of team members and other professionals in patient care.
- How good team working sets direction in order to manage and improve services for patients.
- Clinical team and support services (e.g. nutrition, dietetics, therapists).
- Working relationships of:

  - hospital, primary care and mental health services;
  - hospital and other agencies (e.g. social services, local authority services, police);
  - information transfer from primary to secondary care on admission;
  - the role of the voluntary sector in supporting patients and carers;
  - the principles of providing optimum care within a community setting.

This chapter will also introduce you to the following mandatory level 1 competencies as set out in the generic curriculum for the medical specialties as published by the Federation of the Royal Colleges of Physicians (UK) in 2006.

- Outline the components of effective collaboration.
- Describe the roles and responsibilities of members of the healthcare team.
- Detailed hand over between shifts and areas of care.

Chapter overview

In this chapter, the focus is on teamwork and working collaboratively with both colleagues from one's own profession and other health and social care professionals with whom you come into contact. These professionals may be members of your healthcare team but you will need to work collaboratively with practitioners who are not members of your day-to-day team. The aim is interprofessional collaborative practice with the goal of providing safe and effective patient-centred care.

After reading this chapter you will be able to:

- demonstrate understanding of collaborative and interprofessional approaches to patient care and the benefits to health outcomes of these approaches;
- identify effective and dysfunctional teams and develop strategies for more effective team-working;
- seek out interprofessional learning;
- demonstrate understanding of effective handovers and perform these more effectively.

Context

Twenty-first-century healthcare provision within the UK is dependent on a diverse professional workforce comprising individuals with different roles and responsibilities working within the National Health Service and the private sector. It is rare for any patient to interact with only one health professional during the course of an illness, and certainly patients with chronic conditions will have multiple referrals and interactions for on-going care. Secondary or primary care teams will provide a great part of this care in partnership as well-defined teams with regular meetings, but patients may also access physiotherapists, pharmacists, social workers, psychologists and complementary therapists (to name but a few) who are not necessarily co-located with the rest of the 'team'. This means that communication between professionals and with patients, with an understanding of roles and responsibilities, is of paramount importance to avoid misunderstanding, patients' receiving conflicting messages and no one person having an oversight of the management plan.

The importance of communication between all professionals involved with the same patients was highlighted by the now well-known circumstances that occurred in Bristol, and this case is often referred to as a turning point in patient care. The inquiry into the performance of paediatric heart surgeons in Bristol found that poor communication between different professionals was a factor in the adverse clinical outcomes for the babies involved (Bristol Royal Infirmary Inquiry, 2001). In this hospital setting, the professionals may well have identified that they were working in a team, but other recent high-profile cases, such as that of Baby P, also show a lack of coordinated care across organisations and failure to discuss concerns by the disparate groups of health and social care professionals and agencies involved.

Thus, while many health and social care professionals are not grouped together in 'official' teams while interacting with the same patients, families and carers, the expectation is that they would still take a patient (or client)-centred approach and work collaboratively. Collaborative working is a skill that needs to be learnt, and involves negotiation and often conflict resolution. Most health and social care professionals work within strict boundaries set by their professional bodies and this is sometimes frustrating for others who assume a greater flexibility in patient care. There are hierarchical lines of authority within each profession and different levels of professional autonomy. A doctor may presume to be the clinical leader of a team but then find that a nurse needs to clarify his or her role with someone higher up the nursing hierarchy. Often, health professionals interact individually with patients, setting their own goals and management plans without consultation with others who are involved – a situation which frequently arises due to the fact that patient records are rarely shared (even with the patient).

The interprofessional approach to patient care involves practitioners from different professional backgrounds delivering services and coordinating care programmes to achieve different and often disparate service client needs. Ideally goals are set collaboratively (including with the patient) through consensual decision-making and result in an individualised care plan, which may be delivered by one or more professionals. This level of collaborative practice is difficult to achieve but does maximise the value of shared expertise.

Working and communicating with your team

The European working time directive has led to a change in junior doctors' working patterns so that many are no longer considered to be members of a medical 'firm'. The firm, if it exists, consists of one or more consultants, specialist registrars and foundation doctors, who regularly meet and who care for the same patients. Ward rounds are carried out with nursing staff and ideally everyone is up to date with patient management and treatment goals. Shift patterns of junior doctors may mean that familiarity with other members of staff may be lost, enhancing the need for careful communication and handover.

There are numerous definitions of a team (Box 13.1). Some teams come together for very specific tasks (for example project teams), some change frequently (e.g. as doctors move on to the next stage in their training) and some hardly vary over years (e.g. some practice-based primary care teams). With the patient-centred approach to healthcare, there is also an argument that a patient should be thought of as a member of the team – the patient at the centre of the team.

Box 13.1 Definitions of a team

A team is a small number of people with complementary skills, who are committed to a common purpose, performance, goals and approach, for which they are mutually accountable.

High performance team members are . . . committed to one another (Hammick et al., 2009, p39).

ACTIVITY 13.1 WORKING IN TEAMS

Consider a team of which you are or have been a member. How did this team compare to the definitions given? What helped the team to function well and what could have been improved? What might having a patient as a member of the team look like and what implications does this have for team working?

Hammick et al. (2009) discuss positive ways to behave to enhance team function. These include making sure you have an understanding of the values, knowledge and skills of other team members (especially important if the team includes members from other professions), agreeing ground rules and processes for working together, active participation by all members, listening to each other and engaging in discussions and problem-solving, respecting and maintaining professional relationships, and communicating effectively.

It is important to have self-awareness, to understand your own biases and prejudices to others – these may be the result of stereotyping team members based on their profession, their age or even gender. Beware of such stereotyping and prejudice, which often arise from ignorance, as these may ultimately affect patient care.

Collaborative practice

While collaborative practice may be thought of as synonymous with teamwork, I feel that the concept of collaboration acknowledges the fact that not all people working together are members of defined teams.

Box 13.2 Collaborative practice definitions

The World Health Organisation's (WHO) *Framework for Action on Interprofessional Action and Collaborative Practice* (2010) includes the following definitions:

A collaborative practice-ready health worker is someone who has learned how to work in an interprofessional team and is competent to do so.

Collaborative practice happens when multiple health workers from different professional backgrounds work together with patients, families, carers and communities to deliver the highest quality of care. It allows health workers to engage any individual whose skills can help achieve local health goals.

(p9)

ACTIVITY 13.2 PATIENTS WITH COMPLEX CONDITIONS

Reflect on a patient with a complex condition (either a patient you are currently caring for or one you have interacted with in the past). Which other health professionals are likely to be involved in the diagnosis and management of this patient but who you would not consider to be part of your team? For each of these professionals consider:

• how much you know about their role and responsibilities;
• the level of their professional autonomy and to whom they report;
• how you refer to them and the channels of communication between you and them;
• whether they have access to the same patient records as you do;
• whether you, they and the patient have the same goals and expectations;
• how they record their interaction with 'your' patient;
• whether you have ever interacted with them face to face;
• how you could better collaborate with them to improve patient care.

From your answers to these questions, reflect on whether they demonstrate best practice. If not, how might patient care be improved? Whose responsibility is it to initiate these improvements? How will you know if matters have improved?

Learning together to work together

The answers to activity 13.2 are likely to indicate that there is very little direct interaction between certain health and social care professionals who are nevertheless responsible for the same patient's management. In practice doctors may have only a basic understanding of the roles of others in the wider healthcare team – yet they send their patients to these people for tests and treatments. Many medical schools now provide their students with interprofessional learning activities to ensure that students from different professional programmes gain an understanding of each other's capabilities and approach to patient care before they begin to work together after qualification. This, indeed, is the rationale behind the Foundation competencies that are listed for this chapter. Interprofessional education (IPE) occurs when two or more professions learn with, from and about each other to improve collaboration and quality of care (CAIPE, 1997). IPE may occur pre-registration or post-registration, and may take place in the classroom, clinical environment, community settings and/or online. Interprofessional learning thus occurs through a variety of activities, of different lengths and intensities, and with different learning outcomes (if indeed these are defined). The broad themes of outcomes (or objectives or competencies) are shown in Box 13.3. How many of these did you have to meet or were assessed on as a medical student? Interprofessional learning (learning together to work together) should also be a feature of post-qualification education but the

Collins evaluation of the Foundation Programme (Collins, 2010) found that 35 per cent of trainees never and 34 per cent rarely had the opportunity to learn with other healthcare professionals such as nurses and physiotherapists.

Box 13.3 Examples of interprofessional learning outcomes

Teamwork

- Knowledge of and skills for (including recognition of importance of common goals).
- Knowledge of, skills for and positive attitudes to collaboration with other health. professionals.
- Leadership issues.
- Assume the roles and responsibilities of *team leader* and team member.
- Barriers to teamwork.
- Being an effective team member.
- Team dynamics and power relationships.

Roles and responsibilities

- Knowledge and understanding of the different roles, responsibilities and expertise of health professionals.
- Knowledge and development of one's own professional role.
- Understanding of role/professional boundaries.
- Being able to challenge misconceptions in relations to roles.

Communication

- Communicate effectively with other health professionals.
- Negotiation and conflict resolution.
- Shared decision-making – with other health professionals, members of team, patient, family.
- Communication at beginning and end of shifts (handover, handoff).
- Awareness of difference in professionals' language.
- Exchange of essential clinical information (health records, through electronic media).

Learning/reflection

- Identification of learning needs in relation to future development in a team.
- Reflect critically on one's own relationship within a team.
- Self-questioning of personal prejudice and stereotyped views.

The patient

- The patient's central role in interprofessional care (patient-focused or centred care).

- Understanding of the service user's perspective (and family/carers).
- Working together and cooperatively in the best interests of the patient.
- Patient safety issues.

Ethical/attitudes

- Acknowledge views and ideas of other professionals.
- Respect.
- Acknowledge that each health professional's views are equally valid and important.

(Adapted from Thistlethwaite and Moran, 2010)

ACTIVITY 13.3 THE WHO FRAMEWORK AND COLLABORATIVE PRACTICE

Download a copy of the WHO framework and read the section on the evidence for collaborative practice and improved health outcomes (summarised in Box 13.4). What is the strength of this evidence? What are its weaknesses? How does this type of presentation differ from a systematic review?

Available at:
www2.rgu.ac.uk/ipe/WHO_report_Interprofessional%20Ed%20Sep2509.pdf

---

What is the evidence? Collaborative practice

The *Framework for Action* from the WHO states that there is now evidence to show that collaborative practice enhances health services and improves health out-comes, particularly for patients with chronic diseases. Such practice also improves patient safety, reduces the length of hospital stay and the number of admissions, increases patient and carer satisfaction and promotes treatment adherence.

Collaboration between teams

The interaction and communication within your own team may be exemplary, but your team will need to collaborate with other individuals and teams, in the same setting or in another location. While now over ten years old, a British study into communication behaviours in a hospital setting still resonates and has implications for current practice. Coiera and Tombs (1998) found several examples of inefficiencies with communication between teams. They give one example of a senior consultant trying to transfer a patient to another doctor's team by involving at least two interme-diaries. Through a mechanism similar to the childhood game of Chinese whispers, the message had become substantially distorted by the time the second consultant received it. While delegation is important in a busy clinical environment, we need to consider the possible consequences of such delegation and ensure that checks are in place to avoid compromising patient care. The 1998 research concluded that health professionals need to consider carefully the effects of their communication behav-iour, particularly what the researchers called *interruptive behaviours*, on their own efficiency and effectiveness as well as on that of others.

The primary–secondary care interface

During a patient's journey there may be multiple crossings of the interface between community and secondary care. This is particularly the case for patients with long-term chronic conditions such as diabetes and arthritis, while patients undergoing cancer management are often under the care of many specialists and other health professionals. Individual patients have different ways of dealing with this. Some regard their hospital physician as the 'person in charge'; others look to their general practitioner as the repository of knowledge about their condition. Increasingly there may also be a nurse specialist who spends most time with the patient and family. How are decisions made and what effect does it have on collaborative working?

Health professionals interacting with patients need to explore with patients (and their carers as appropriate) who is also providing advice and treatment. You may, on eliciting a history on admission, ask about this (not only who the GP is) and explore what the patient understands about the roles of these professionals and how they interact. Just as it is common to ignore inquiring about over the counter and comple-mentary medicines, it is likely that often you will forget to ask about complementary therapists and community-based healthcare professionals. Doctors need to explore what patients understand about their condition (ideas and concerns) and where they have gained such information (perhaps the Internet, but it could be their midwife, the community psychiatric nurse, the osteopath). It soon becomes apparent that not only do these clinicians use different language and concepts to describe illness and disease mechanisms, but also that the patient filters and makes sense of this lan-guage, fitting new information into existing health beliefs, which are also affected by the patient's values. If a doctor dismisses this knowledge from the patient's trusted sources, even denigrates it either verbally or through body language, the patient–doctor relationship will get off to a bad start, and the patient may not listen to the doctor's information and advice.

A doctor's values affect communication, though we might not always be aware of this. If I think that osteopathy is 'quackery' and a waste of money, I am unlikely to consider any positive therapeutic effect that the patient describes as important. Patients recognise this scepticism and may be reluctant to talk about such interven-tions in the future. They may even dismiss the orthodox treatment advocated by their doctors and not adhere to management plans as they conflict with what they already believe.

The same problems may arise when discussing patients with other professionals (this takes place commonly on the phone rather than face to face). There may be language barriers (due to professional jargon), conflicting values and mismatch in knowledge about a patient's circumstances. For example, a social worker or occupational therapist may have visited a patient at home and seen difficulties with the neighbourhood that prevent the patient getting about easily and safely, yet the doctor may advise regular outdoor exercise as he only sees the patient in the outpatient clinic.

Optimal collaboration

We may apply theoretical and practical knowledge about teams to other forms of collaboration between health and social care professionals. Researchers at Aston University have described three conditions necessary for functioning teamwork, which may be adapted for collaborative practice (Box 13.5) (Dawson et al., 2007).

Box 13.4 Conditions for functioning teamwork

- Clear objectives that are known to all members – these will be framed in terms of patient goals and should be defined in partnership with the patient.
- Team members work closely together to achieve these objectives – need to think what working closely together means if collaborators are spread over different locations.
- Regular meetings to review team effectiveness and discuss how it can be improved – this does not always happen in well-defined healthcare teams and would be very rare indeed that other collaborators would meet face to face.

ACTIVITY 13.4 EFFECTIVE HANDOVER

Consider the three conditions in Box 13.5. When you hand over a patient to another team, either in the hospital, from the hospital to primary care or primary care to the hospital, in what ways can you ensure that the new team is aware of the goals that you and your patient have set? If the patient will return to your care, how do you collaborate with the new team and continue to do your best for your patient? If you can't meet with the new team after handover, how do you ensure quality care and communication between yourself, the patients and the new team?

Handover

The handover of patients from one team to another has been defined as an important workforce competence within the NHS. The reduction in the number of hours worked by junior doctors, increasing shift patterns and less well-defined clinical firms have all led to the number of occasions on which patient care is transferred. Handover commonly takes place at the end of shift, or when patients are transferred from one specialty to another either within the same hospital or to a different healthcare setting. The transfer may be permanent or temporary. Compared to nursing, shift-to-shift handover amongst medical staff is not a well- defined process. Interdisciplinary or interprofessional handover is much less common. The handover process shifts responsibility for the patient's care to the new team and may be carried out face to face, on the telephone and/or in writing (paper and/or electronically). All three of these methods have advantages and disadvantages, but which one is used is usually necessitated by the particular circumstances.

Patient transfer should take place within normal working hours if possible, unless for emergency reasons. Certainly if a patient is being discharged back home, the GP needs to be informed; this is less feasible after hours. The next of kin/carer/family need to be aware of any location change and indeed this should have been discussed prior to the change, if possible. The clinician doing the handover needs to check that the information about the patient has been understood by the new team member(s), including drug dosages, allergies and other ongoing treatment.

What's the evidence? Handover

Poorly performed clinical handover has implications for patient safety and can lead to poor continuity of care, adverse events and even litigation (Wong et al., 2008). Face-to-face handover, particularly if interprofessional, gives an opportunity for professionals to interact and potentially learn from each other. However, verbal handover only, compared to verbal handover with some written notes, relies heavily on memory and is therefore a high-risk strategy (Bhabra et al., 2007). One study of doctors' performance on simulated handover cycles showed that only a third of the information given was remembered after the first handover cycle and, more concerning, only 2.5 per cent of information was retained after five handover cycles (Pothier et al., 2005). If carried out face to face or via telephone, written notes should be made about what has been said, what instructions given and agreed goals. Using prepared sheets, with spaces for appropriate information, ensured that the correct information was given and retained (Pothier et al., 2005).

ACTIVITY 13.5

This builds on activity 13.4 but is more practical. In your own clinical setting, consider the process of patient handover. Have you ever received any training in this?

- *If yes*: was the training helpful? Did it reflect actual practice? Consider how the training could be improved.
- *If no*: devise a training session on handover, which should also have improving handover as one objective.

Improving training could be based on an audit of the handover procedures in your clinical setting. How would you go about conducting such an audit?

A training session could involve a role play – ask colleagues, preferably from other professions, to work with you. Practise handing over a patient in pairs, with a third person observing and then giving feedback.

Dysfunctional collaboration

Considering Box 13.5 again, Dawson et al. (2007) found that those health professionals who identified themselves as working in teams but who did not meet all three of the parameters shown reported less job satisfaction and more burnout. There were also issues with patient safety if the team was dysfunctional.

Collaboration might disintegrate for a number of reasons. There needs to be a designated coordinator of tasks. There may be personal disagreements between collaborators. Obviously personal feelings should not affect professional duties. However, we are all human and such feelings can lead to poor clinical and interpersonal performance and subsequent stress, with the potential of affecting the morale of others and patient care.

Junior doctors may have difficulties in interacting with their senior colleagues in other teams, particularly if these seniors are not open to suggestion and feedback. Juniors are often unable to challenge the views or actions of their superiors, even if they attempt to do so in a respectful way. Senior doctors and/or other healthcare professionals have been known to resort to bullying, or even they may find it difficult to give feedback constructively on poor performance, leaving such behaviour unchecked. As health professionals ascend the hierarchy, they do not always receive training in leadership or personnel management. They may be unable to delegate or mentor juniors in a supportive and educational manner (Thistlethwaite and Spencer, 2009).

Dysfunctional teams may be helped by team meetings, sometimes with outside consultants, to build team morale and diagnose difficulties. However, such remediation is difficult for people who collaborate but who do not work in the same team, as often there is no mechanism to deal with these interrelationships.

Case study 13.1: Working with colleagues

John Rigg is a F1 doctor working for four months with the gastroen-terology team. His in-patients are mainly located on four wards. He is finding it difficult to get on with the charge nurse of one of these wards. The nurse bleeps him a lot more than the other nurses he works with, and criticises him for taking his time, the way he talks to patients and how he fills in the notes. John has not had any negative feedback from other colleagues. Today his registrar Sue tells him that the charge nurse has complained to her about John's attitude.

What is the best way of dealing with this situation?

Case study reflection

This is obviously a difficult situation for both John and Sue. First, John needs to know exactly what the charge nurse has said about him, and whether Sue has any reservations about his work. It would also be useful to know Sue's impression of the charge nurse and whether he is prone to making criticisms. John then needs to reflect on his performance to decide if he does need to improve. A multisource feedback might be helpful. If John feels that the charge nurse's complaint is unfounded, he should ask to speak to him, preferably with Sue and/or another nurse present, to discuss the issues. John and the charge nurse should both be working towards the best out-comes for their shared patients and such a dispute will affect John's work, and his collaboration with a nursing colleagues. It might also affect his view of nurses, with long-term negative consequences. He needs to adopt measures to resolve the conflict by communicating with the nurse in a non-threatening and open way, showing he is ready to learn and change if necessary, but also to defend himself against erroneous impressions.

What to do when things go wrong

There are a number of scenarios to consider as there are so many different profes-sionals and support staff with whom you may interact, including peers and senior staff. You may also be supervising or mentoring juniors – for example, medical stu-dents – for whom you may be responsible for part of the day. You should be aware of lines of responsibility and whom to ask for advice if difficulties arise. Your mentor or educational supervisor should be able to help if your immediate clinical superior is not available. Of course, dealing with the matter by speaking to whomever is trou-bling you is always the best way to start the process, but this may not be possible face to face or you may be overpowered by their position. Sometimes difficult working relationships are due to simple misunderstandings and poor communication. Remember that many people you do come into contact with are more permanent in their positions, while you will rotate frequently in the workplace. You may inadvertently go against convention and you may be judged against previous doctors in your position. Chapters 3, 17 and 18 provide some ideas of how you might work with others more effectively and 'stress proof' yourself.

Of course it is always better to avoid conflict by working courteously and by showing respect. You should also expect that if you work in this way, you should also be treated with respect. Introduce yourself by name and designation. The colleagues around you should know the limits of your experience, your role and responsibilities, but may need reminding in tense situations. You need to research the roles and responsibilities of your colleagues, and if this is not covered in orientation, you should ask for clarification if you have any uncertainty.

Chapter summary

- The importance of communication and team-working skills cannot be over-emphasised in the twenty-first-century health service.

- However, collaboration with colleagues from one's own and other professions, who are not part of the day-to-day team, is extremely important.

- Knowing roles and responsibilities, involving the patient in decisions, communication between all involved in a patient's care and negotiation skills are all important for ensuring good practice, optimal outcomes and patient safety.

GOING FURTHER

Getting started: an introduction and overview **www.rcn.org.uk/__data/assets/ pdf_file/0003/78735/003115.pdf**
This links to documents on developing and sustaining effective teams and draws on evidence in relation to what a team is, effective roles, team meetings, dealing with conflict, and change and transition.

A useful resource about handover is Australian: the OSSIE guide to clinical handover improvement (2010), available at: **www.health.gov.au/internet/safety/ publishing.nsf/content/PriorityProgram-05_OssieGuide/$FILE/ossie. pdf**

Information about pilot projects relating to handover in the UK is available at: **www.healthcareworkforce.nhs.uk/teamworkinghandoverandescalation. html**

Leadership and Management Skills
Judy McKimm

Achieving foundation competences

This chapter will help you to begin to meet the following requirements of the *Foundation Programme Curriculum* (2010).

Outcome 1 Professionalism

- Practise with professionalism including: integrity; compassion; altruism; continuous improvement; aspiration to excellence; respect of cultural and ethnic diversity; regard to the principles of equity; ethical behaviour; probity (refer to GMC *Fitness to Practise* declaration in F1 and *Standards for Training for the Foundation Programme* in *The New Doctor*); leadership.

Outcome 14 Working with colleagues

- Demonstrates effective teamwork skills within the clinical team and in the larger medical context.

14.1 Communication with colleagues and teamwork for patient safety

Knowledge

- F1 – displays understanding of personal role within the team and is able to support a team leader; listens to views of other healthcare professionals; takes leadership role and delegates appropriately in the context of own competence; demonstrates awareness of local major incident planning and their potential role in any such incident; meticulously cross-checks instructions and actions with colleagues (e.g. medicines to be injected); describes ways of identifying and dealing with poor performance in self and in colleagues.

- F2 – shows leadership skills where appropriate and at the same time works effectively with others towards a common goal.

14.2 Interface with different specialties and with other professionals

- F1 – shows an understanding of the challenges of providing optimum care within a variety of clinical settings; arranges appropriate urgent investigations and chases results when necessary.

- F2 – consistently seeks effective communication with colleagues in other disciplines; describes the process of referral from primary to secondary care.

The chapter will also introduce you to the leadership and management outcomes set out in the *Compendium of Academic Competencies* published by the UK Foundation Programme Office; the *Medical Leadership Competency Framework* (Academy of Medical Royal Colleges and the NHS Institute for Innovation and Improvement, 2010) and *Management for Doctors* (General Medical Council).

Chapter overview

> Leadership is not an esoteric topic relevant to a select few, but a ubiquitous feature of daily life for every physician.
>
> (Gunderman, 2009)

Effective clinical leadership and management is vital for ensuring that health services run effectively and efficiently, that all members of the healthcare team work well together and that patient care and safety is improved. Clinical leadership and management activities operate at all levels, from managing a clinical situation at the bedside through to balancing the budget of a large NHS trust. It is not always easy for medical students and junior doctors to see where they might fit into the large bureaucracy of the NHS (the NHS 'supertanker'), and more difficult still to see what sort of leadership or management role might be appropriate. This chapter explores what is meant by clinical leadership and management and how foundation doctors might participate in these activities.

After reading this chapter you will be able to:

- discuss the key features of clinical leadership and management;
- identify how you might improve your own clinical practice;
- apply leadership approaches and management tools to clinical situations;
- identify areas for service improvement.

Introduction

The importance of effective leadership and management in healthcare has been the focus of international attention for decades. Public health services take a large amount of taxpayers' money and are one of the main draws on the public purse. As technological and pharmaceutical advances come into the public domain, expectations from the health service (from both those who use and deliver the service) grow year on year. With around 1.4 million employees, the UK National Health Service (NHS) is the fourth largest civilian employer in the world. It is not possible to manage an organisation of this size centrally. Managing this huge enterprise and delivering safe, high-quality patient care at point of use requires strong, clear leadership from government with a devolved management and leadership structure.

Over the last decade, we have seen a shift from the NHS being managed by 'professional' managers, the majority of whom did not have clinical backgrounds, to a mixed model where non-clinical managers work alongside clinical managers to deliver the service. One reason that this came about was to address the widening divide between managers and clinicians. Managers were typically seen as target driven, budget focused and not appreciative of the complexities of delivering high-quality patient care. Doctors were seen as subverting management decisions and failing to understand the need to work towards targets and keep to budgets. Management was seen as 'the dark side'. These stereotypes were not only unhelpful, but also did not reflect the reality of many experienced clinicians and managers who worked together in harmony. However, increasing calls were being made to address these issues and engage doctors more actively in leadership (Imison and Giordano, 2009)

What's the evidence? Involving doctors in leadership

A large body of evidence has been gathered internationally that demonstrates that the involvement of doctors in leadership and management influences organisational performance and improves health outcomes for patients. A summary of the international literature on medical engagement can be found in the NHS Institute for Innovation and Improvement and Academy of Medical Royal Colleges papers:

- *Engaging Doctors in Leadership: what can we learn from international experience and research evidence?* (2008a)
- *Engaging Doctors: can doctors influence organizational performance?* (2008b)

In the UK, many bodies have been working together to identify what clinical leadership and management means in practice and how health professionals can be trained and supported in their leadership roles. For doctors, a specific direction has been taken in the development of the *Medical Leadership Competency Framework* (MLCF, 2010, Academy of Medical Royal Colleges and the NHS Institute for Innovation and Improvement) which provides a set of competencies and guidance around developing leadership for medical students, postgraduate trainees and doctors in continuing practice, see Figure 14.1.

The MLCF is supported by a series of e-learning modules called LeAD for postgraduate trainees and clinical tutors (**www.e-lfh.org.uk/lead**). The General Medical Council (GMC) also sets out leadership requirements in *Tomorrow's Doctors* (2009a), *Good Medical Practice* (2006) and *Management for Doctors* (2006a) which have incorporated ideas from the MLCF. And the 58 specialty training curricula of the Medical Royal Colleges and Faculties have also integrated the MLCF. We have therefore used the framework as the basis for structuring this chapter as you will encounter this in practice and can utilise the additional resources available to enhance and extend your understanding of leadership.

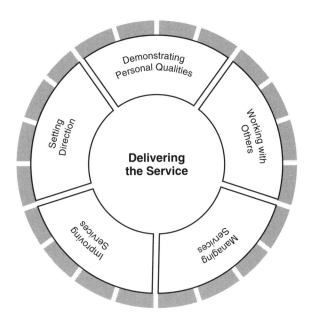

Figure 14.1 The Medical Leadership Competency Framework 2010, Academy of Medical Royal Colleges and the NHS Institute for Innovation and Improvement, ©NHS Institute for Innovation and Improvement and Academy of Royal Medical Colleges 2010. All rights reserved. Reproduced with permission.**www.institute.nhs.uk/ assessment_tool/general/medical_leadership_competency_framework_- _homepage.html**

Leadership and management: Theory to practice

> Before the start of the programme, I was very naive to the idea of clinical leadership. The idea had never been discussed in medical school. Once I had graduated and started working, the idea was rarely discussed. When it was discussed, it was not for my benefit.
>
> (F2 leader)

Leadership theory provides us with many models and approaches which have been applied throughout the last 50 or 60 years. Although new models seem to emerge almost monthly, it is not that one model should be seen as replacing another as a 'truth' but rather that each model gives us a different way of looking at leadership in various situations or contexts. They should be seen as a way of explaining what is going on or as a means of developing behaviours for different situations and not as a strict recipe for action.

One of the challenges for medical students and junior doctors is that leadership and management are not simply activities that are done in practice, but that they are underpinned by subject disciplines with bodies of theory in their own right. These disciplines are not typically studied at medical school and beyond, although this is changing. The language and terms used are drawn primarily from social sciences and much of the evidence is gathered using qualitative methodologies. This can feel quite off-putting to medics who are more used to scientific terminology and quantitative methods of seeking evidence. As we go through the chapter, we will provide some core theory to explain practical situations, taking each of the domains in the MLCF in turn to discuss how leadership theory might help to inform your practice.

Managing services

Management and leadership were traditionally seen as different and separate. Management is often seen as about stability, maintaining the status quo and organising resources whereas leadership is seen as about change, enacting vision, setting direction, influencing others and aligning people. However, although there is some credence to this separation, an effective organisation actually needs both and, increasingly, leadership and management are seen as two sides of the same coin. In organisations with hierarchical structures, most doctors will be appointed to management roles (e.g. medical director or head of department or service) which have both management and leadership responsibilities. An organisation or department that is over-managed may slide into mediocrity and whilst it may meet targets, balance budgets and be well organised, there is little room for innovation and change. On the other hand, without effective management, there may be no money spare to carry out the innovations or changes that are envisaged, or the right people may not be in place to take forward the changes. A good leader therefore pays attention to both aspects, either through forming a team that has all the right skills or acquiring those skills themselves. Figure 14.2 sets out the MLCF areas within the 'managing services' domain.

At foundation stage, it is unlikely that your leadership will be around leading or managing a department but that your leadership activities will be centred more around leading in the clinical context or through participation in projects. Let's take a clinical example.

Case study 14.1: Clinical leadership at the bedside

You are the F2 who is called to a ward to see a patient who has severe chest pain. You are working with a nurse and there are no other doctors free. As you are examining the patient, they suddenly arrest. As the only doctor there, you take an immediate leadership role and quickly think about who else needs to be there (aligning people), what clinical protocols need to be followed (clinical management) and what needs to be done to meet resuscitation guidance and patient's needs (issuing instructions, working with others, practical tasks).

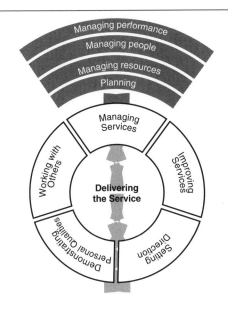

The MLCF (2010, pp42–51) suggests that doctors need to demonstrate competence in the areas of:

- Planning: actively contributing to plans to achieve service goals.

- Managing resources: knowing what resources are available and using their influence to ensure that resources are used efficiently and safely, and reflect the diversity of needs.

- Managing people: providing direction, reviewing performance, motivating others, and promoting equality and diversity.

- Managing performance: holding themselves and others accountable for service outcomes.

The Medical Leadership Competency Framework, 2010, Academy of Medical Royal Colleges and the NHS Institute for Innovation and Improvement,
© NHS Institute for Innovation and Improvement and Academy of Royal Medical Colleges 2010. All rights reserved. Reproduced with permission.
www.institute.nhs.uk/assessment_tool/ general/managing_services.html

Figure 14.2 Managing services

This illustrates how a combination of leadership and management skills are required in relatively routine clinical scenarios. As you become more experienced, this will all seem to happen intuitively, but in the early stages 'novice' doctors tend to focus on the practical tasks, with the 'non-technical skills' (communication, leadership, etc.) having to be thought through. The benefit of de-briefing and feedback after real or simulated clinical situations can help you recognise your impact on others and develop your leadership skills alongside your clinical competence.

Medical students and foundation trainees can also learn to develop organisational awareness and understand more about management systems, structures and cultures in their own and others' workplaces. This not only helps you deliver a better service to your patients and work more effectively with colleagues but can also help you to identify areas or issues with which you might want to engage more actively. All healthcare organisations have ongoing projects which include aspects of service redesign, audit and health improvement initiatives. To help you be more effective in audit and other projects, acquiring some basic project management techniques and management tools might be useful, see Box 14.1.

Two helpful web resources that will help you learn more about these and the wide range of other techniques are the NHS Institute for Innovation and Improvement

---

Box 14.1 Examples of management tools and techniques

SWOT analysis – this tool considers the internal Strengths and Weaknesses of an organisation, department or team and the external Opportunities and Threats. Once the analysis has been carried out, then a plan can be made as to how to build on the strengths and seize opportunities and address weaknesses and minimise or work around threats.

PESTLE (or PEST or PESTELI) analysis – this is used for analysis of external factors or forces that might impact on the organisation, department or team. These are the Political, Economic, Socio-demographic, Technological, Legal and Environmental factors. Like the SWOT analysis, PESTLE helps you to carry out a structured analysis and then devise an action plan to address the impact of the various factors.

---

website (**www.institute.nhs.uk**), which includes videos, tools, techniques, ideas and case examples of 'innovation', 'safer care' and 'quality and value', and the JISC Infokits site (**www.jiscinfonet.ac.uk/infokits**), which includes information on 'project management', 'change management' and 'tools and techniques'.

Working with others

The focus on 'medical leadership' taken by the MLCF moves away from the more generic term 'clinical leadership and management' which includes all clinicians (nurses, physiotherapists, etc.). However, the MLCF does include aspects of management and rationalises its focus on medical leadership by noting that 'all doctors work within systems and within organisations. It is a vitally important fact that doctors have a direct and far-reaching impact on patient experience and outcomes. Doctors have a legal duty broader than any other health professional and therefore have an intrinsic leadership role within healthcare services' (2010, p6). Notwithstanding the key role doctors play in patient care and health services, it is important that doctors do not simply assume leadership without recognising the roles played by others in multidisciplinary teams or the wider organisation and being able to demonstrate the skills and understanding to lead effectively. Assuming leadership without paying attention to some of the competences and issues we explore in this chapter, could lead to perceptions of arrogance from others and, at worst, a clinical disaster. Chapters 6, 7 and 13 discuss the importance of communication and non-technical skills in ensuring patient safety.

As mentioned earlier in the chapter, the different models of leadership are underpinned by a body of leadership theory, which is in itself drawn from a range of perspectives primarily from the social sciences. The MLCF emphasises a model of 'shared leadership' 'where leadership is not restricted to people who hold designated leadership roles and where there is a shared sense of responsibility for the success of the organisation and its services. Acts of leadership can come from anyone in the organisation, as appropriate at different times, and are focused on the achievement of the group rather than of an individual. Thus shared leadership actively supports effective teamwork' (2010, p6). The model of 'shared leadership' has much in common with other models of leadership, including collaborative leadership and dispersed or distributed leadership.

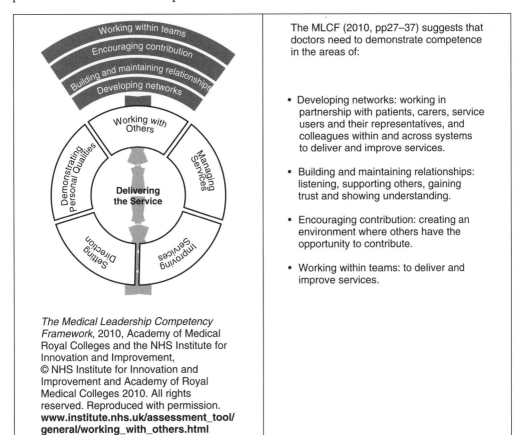

The MLCF (2010, pp27–37) suggests that doctors need to demonstrate competence in the areas of:

- Developing networks: working in partnership with patients, carers, service users and their representatives, and colleagues within and across systems to deliver and improve services.

- Building and maintaining relationships: listening, supporting others, gaining trust and showing understanding.

- Encouraging contribution: creating an environment where others have the opportunity to contribute.

- Working within teams: to deliver and improve services.

The Medical Leadership Competency Framework, 2010, Academy of Medical Royal Colleges and the NHS Institute for Innovation and Improvement, © NHS Institute for Innovation and Improvement and Academy of Royal Medical Colleges 2010. All rights reserved. Reproduced with permission. **www.institute.nhs.uk/assessment_tool/ general/working_with_others.html**

Figure 14.3 Working with others

Clinical situations you will be involved with include case conferences, multi-disciplinary discharge planning and formulating and implementing care plans in collaboration with other members of the interdisciplinary team.

Demonstrating personal qualities

Early approaches to explaining leadership emphasised the importance of personality traits and personal qualities such as integrity, consistency and charisma. Such 'great man' theories provided us with a way of viewing leaders as individuals in whom the responsibility and reward for leadership was invested. Great military leaders, explorers, prime ministers and presidents are often, even today, valued for their personal leadership qualities (as 'charismatic leaders') as well as for their actions.

The qualities valued in leaders reflect the dominant values and beliefs of the time as well as the cultures in which leadership is exercised and leaders can (if they do not respond to change) become out of step and 'time expired'. Also, if leaders are given too much power and control, the individual 'hero' leader can (if they do not have self-control and insight) lead a team, organisation or country into very risky territory.

Although personality-based or 'trait' theories need to be applied with some care, the idea that personal qualities and behaviours are important to leadership is still very pervasive and, indeed, who would want to be led by a doctor who did not display integrity, professional values and compassion? The idea of 'ethical' or 'value-led' leadership is highly pertinent to medical leadership, which relies on the sanctity of the doctor–patient relationship and an adherence to the highest professional standards as set out in *Good Medical Practice* (GMC, 2006). In Chapter 3, you read about the importance of understanding yourself, learning about how your personality and behaviours impact on and influence others. Demonstrating personal qualities that people associate with leadership are vitally important if you are to manage clinical teams or projects and, as you get more senior, lead departments or organisations. Figure 14.4 sets out what the MLCF defines as core personal qualities.

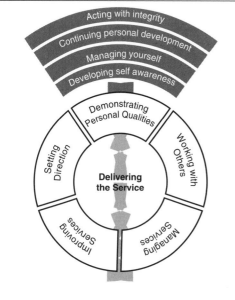

The MLCF (2010, pp14–23) suggests that doctors need to demonstrate competence in the areas of:

- Developing self-awareness: being aware of their own values, principles and assumptions and being able to learn from experiences.

- Managing yourself: organising and managing themselves while taking account of the needs and priorities of others.

- Continuing personal development (CPD): learning through participating in CPD and from experience and feedback.

- Acting with integrity: behaving in an open, honest and ethical manner.

The Medical Leadership Competency Framework, 2010, Academy of Medical Royal Colleges and the NHS Institute for Innovation and Improvement,
© NHS Institute for Innovation and Improvement and Academy of Royal Medical Colleges 2010. All rights reserved. Reproduced with permission.
www.institute.nhs.uk/assessment_tool/ general/demonstrating_personal_ qualities.html

Figure 14.4 Demonstrating personal qualities

Greenleaf's (1977) model of 'servant leadership' (first evolved from church leadership) suggests that leaders in public service aspire to serve first and then to aspire to lead. In other words, doctors may initially want to make a difference to individual patients and their care but, as they realise that in order to make more effective and long-lasting changes, they need to influence health organisations and systems, they then aspire to move into a leadership role. The idea that leaders might not simply be 'born' (i.e. genetically predisposed to behaviours associated with leadership) but that leadership can be learned has influenced many theorists and underpins leadership development programmes. For example, Goleman's concept of 'emotional intelligence' (2000) suggests that being aware of your own strengths and limitations and thus being able to self-regulate your behaviours is a marker of being able to work well with others and lead effectively.

ACTIVITY 14.1 EMOTIONAL INTELLIGENCE

Cherniss and Goleman (2001) in The Emotionally Intelligent Workplace suggest that emotional intelligence (EQ) can be learned and can improve leadership behaviours. They categorise the components of EQ into four areas: those concerned with recognition and regulation and those concerned with your own personal competence (knowing yourself and managing yourself appropriately) and your social competence (being aware of how you work with others and controlling and managing how you work with others).

Taking the lists in each of the four boxes below, try to identify what you think are your strengths and areas for development. Discuss this with a colleague, ideally another foundation doctor, and compare notes. This activity should provide you with some feedback on your own emotional intelligence and identify areas for development or further learning.

	Self (Personal Competence)	*Other (Social Competence)*
Recognition	**Self-awareness** • Emotional self-awareness • Accurate self-assessment • Self-confidence	**Social awareness** • Empathy • Service orientation • Organisational awareness
Regulation	**Self-management** • Emotional self control • Trustworthiness • Conscientiousness • Adaptability • Achievement drive • Initiative	**Relationship management** • Developing others • Influence • Communication • Conflict management • Visionary leadership • Catalysing change • Building bonds • Teamwork and collaboration

The relationship between professional practice and identity and leadership behaviours and role is one that every doctor will need to explore and develop for themselves (see Chapter 3). Another set of theories consider leadership behaviours and the ways in which leaders needed to focus on achieving a balance between the task, the team and the individual (Adair, 1973) or between concern for task and concern for people (Blake and Mouton, 1964). 'Contingency theories' suggest that leaders have to employ different styles and strategies to meet the demands of different situations. There is no one leadership style that works for all contexts, leadership is 'situational' and leaders need to be able to use 'multiple styles seamlessly' (Yukl, 2002). In the clinical context, you will need to take a different leadership style if there is an emergency (where an authoritative or command and control style may well be relevant) from chairing a case conference with a multidisciplinary team. In the latter situation, a more effective style may be much more participatory, affiliative or democratic, with a need for facilitating discussions to enable joint decision-making.

The relationship between leadership and management can be seen in models of leadership such as transactional leadership or 'reward-exchange theory' where leadership is seen as based on a series of transactions between the organisation and those who work in it. Whilst leaders need to be able to motivate those who work for or with them (and of course pay and conditions of work are part of this), the relationship between leaders and 'followers' is more complex than a simple exchange of labour for some reward. Studies on followership emphasise the importance of leaders being able to both lead and follow. Kelley (1992), for example, suggests that in any situation we may choose to take one of four leadership or followership roles: passive followership; active followership; little 'l' leadership; and big 'L' leadership. One way of becoming more aware of possibilities for your own leadership role is to seek opportunities for different ways of leading and following. For example, whilst participating in ward rounds, in theatre or in out-patient clinics, look at situations where you might become more active, as a 'follower' (where a senior is clearly taking the lead but where you are actively involved in providing information, examining patients or in practical procedures under direction) or as you move into a little 'l' leadership role and require less supervision or direction. Here you might take a business ward round or teach medical students, close a wound or lead some out-patient clinic activities. It is unlikely that you will move into big 'L' leadership as a foundation doctor but you can start preparing for such future roles.

Improving services

The final models of leadership that are very influential in considering how organisations manage through change are those of transformational leadership and complex adaptive leadership. Transformational leadership emerged as a response to the more transactional approaches discussed above which failed to help organisations survive and flourish in times of rapid external change (Bass and Avolio, 1994). This concept has been very influential in the NHS and underpins the ideas of shared leadership set out in the MLCF. We discuss this and complex adaptive leadership more fully in the next section.

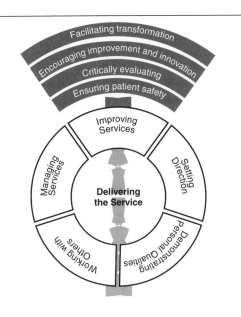

The MLCF (2010, pp56–65) suggests that doctors need to demonstrate competence in the areas of:

- Ensuring patient safety: assessing and managing the risk to patients associated with service developments, balancing economic considerations with the need for patient safety.

- Critically evaluating: being able to think analytically, conceptually and to identify where services can be improved, working individually or as part of a team.

- Encouraging improvement and innovation: creating a climate of continuous service improvement.

- Facilitating transformation: actively contributing to change processes that lead to improving healthcare.

The Medical Leadership Competency Framework, 2010, Academy of Medical Royal Colleges and the NHS Institute for Innovation and Improvement, © NHS Institute for Innovation and Improvement and Academy of Royal Medical Colleges 2010. All rights reserved. Reproduced with permission. **www.institute.nhs.uk/assessment_tool/ general/setting_direction.html**

Figure 14.5 Improving services

What's the evidence? 'Lean thinking'

An example of service improvement that has been employed in health services around the world is that of lean management or 'lean thinking'. Lean management principles have been used effectively in manufacturing for decades and are based around the ideas of reducing waste (of time, goodwill, money or supplies/ equipment), improving flow and adding value to the customer (or patient or other workers) at all steps in complex processes (Institute of Health Improvement, 2005).

A realist literature review of the literature on lean thinking in healthcare (Mazzocatto et al., 2010) concluded that lean thinking has been applied successfully in a wide variety of healthcare settings. Although lean theory emphasises a holistic view, most cases report narrower technical applications with limited organisational reach. They found that common contextual aspects interact with different components of the lean interventions to trigger four change mechanisms: raising awareness and understanding of processes to generate a shared understanding; organising and designing systems and processes for effectiveness and efficiency; improving error detection to increase awareness and process reliability; and collaborating to systematically solve problems to enhance continual improvement. 'To better realise the potential benefits, healthcare organisations need to directly involve senior management, work across functional divides, pursue value creation for patients and other customers, and nurture a long-term view of continual improvement' (Mazzocatto et al., 2010 p376).

ACTIVITY 14.2 DEVELOPING AWARENESS

Start to make yourself more aware of key policy and strategy change drivers and become involved with discussions or initiatives in which the organisation or department is responding to external demands or policies. Depending on where you work, there will be many examples of policy agendas (such as GP commissioning, reduced waiting targets, national service frameworks, impact of long-term conditions strategy) being implemented at local level.

It is useful also to be aware of how tools and techniques (such as audit, clinical governance, lean management processes and systems re-engineering and redesign) are being used in the workplace. The NHS Institute website has interesting examples of case studies of successful and unsuccessful change improvement initiatives.

Setting direction

In transformational leadership, 'followers' are motivated by leaders raising them to higher aspirations and human potential is released through empowerment and development. Vision and values are clearly stated and the organisation and the work of individuals within it are aligned to the achievement of longer-term goals. One of the core qualities defined in most leadership models (and one which is often differentiated from management skills) is the ability to inspire people through setting and communicating a vision.

Tools and techniques that you may need to be more aware of include strategic management, setting objectives, horizon scanning, policy analysis and visioning. As in Activity 14.2 above, start to be more actively aware of the healthcare policies being discussed in the media or in the workplace. Observe how people or organisations use metaphor and other tools for communicating vision.

In many of the models we have discussed, leadership is dispersed and undertaken 'at all levels'. More recently, systems and complexity theory have become

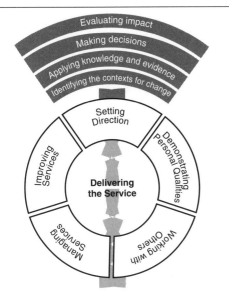

The MLCF (2010, pp70–79) suggests that doctors need to demonstrate competence in the areas of:

- Identifying the contexts for change: being aware of the range of factors to be taken into account.

- Applying knowledge and evidence: gathering information to produce an evidence-based challenge to systems and processes in order to identify opportunities for service improvements.

- Making decisions: using their values, and the evidence, to make good decisions.

- Evaluating impact: measuring and evaluating outcomes, taking corrective action where necessary and by being held to account for their decisions.

The Medical Leadership Competency Framework, 2010, Academy of Medical Royal Colleges and the NHS Institute for Innovation and Improvement, © NHS Institute for Innovation and Improvement and Academy of Royal Medical Colleges 2010. All rights reserved. Reproduced with permission. **www.institute.nhs.uk/assessment_tool/ general/setting_direction.html**

Figure 14.6 Setting direction

influential in considering how organisations cope with and adapt to change (Plsek and Greenhalgh, 2001; Kernick, 2010). The leader's role as 'change agent' is one that distinguishes a leader from a manager, and is a core leadership activity. The dominant leadership model here is 'complex adaptive leadership' where the leader is consciously working within a complex system, aware of its component parts and how these work together, working flexibly and responsively to internal and external change and ensuring that the organisation, department or team remains in a state of readiness for responding positively to change. Complexity theory offers ideas such as how introducing or changing 'simple rules' (i.e. the four hour waiting time target in emergency departments) have massive organisational impact and allow change to be emergent as long as boundaries are clearly set. The leaders' role is to hold the boundaries and ensure that the system is not allowed to fall into chaos.

Of course, it is difficult and often inappropriate for students or junior doctors to engage in setting direction and managing services at whole system level, but there are many examples where junior doctors are engaging meaningfully in leadership activities. The case study below describes one such initiative.

Case study 14.2: The Leicester Academic Programme in Clinical Leadership and Management

A unique academic clinical leadership and management programme commenced in Leicester in 2009 for 12 F2 doctors working in the Emergency Medicine department. All trainees took a Postgraduate Certificate in Clinical Leadership and Management at the University of Leicester. As part of the programme, all trainees carried out a leadership project and worked with tutors on a research project to identify what 'junior doctor leadership' is all about. What they realised early on was that medical school had not prepared them for a more formal leadership role and that the applied leadership and management theory was vital. At the end of the programme they summed up their messages to other foundation trainees.

Junior doctors can contribute to clinical leadership and management by:

- working on small-scale health innovation projects, collecting evidence and analysing data and acting as project champions;
- bringing a fresh perspective and ideas to clinical problems and issues;
- providing momentum and energy;
- building bridges between different stakeholders;
- providing feedback to other junior doctors from the wider context;
- carrying out management activities such as options appraisals, SWOT analyses, etc.;
- observing practice;
- taking a team leader and member role;
- making suggestions, but not taking decisions;
- identifying needs;
- influencing small-scale change.

The key knowledge, skills and values and behaviours that they think junior doctors need in terms of leadership and management are set out in Table 14.1.

Knowledge	Skills and behaviours	Values
• Clinical knowledge	• Strategic thinking	• Dedication
• Leadership and management theory and knowledge	• Time management	• Integrity
	• Good communication	• Abundance mentality
	• Conflict management and being able to	• Valuing others,

- ○ Awareness of leadership styles

- NHS policy, strategy. structure and systems
- Situational awareness and understanding of the organisation
- Change management
- Project management

minimise resistance
- Emotional intelligence
  - ○ Empathy
  - ○ Personal awareness and insight

- Peer support
- Analytical skills
- Negotiation and influencing skills
- Networking
- A tactful approach
- Resilience and patience
- Positivity, self motivation and being proactive
- Being interested

especially non-doctors and managers
- High-quality patient care and safety

Their key messages to other foundation trainees thinking of taking an academic programme in leadership and management were:

- It is a positive experience.
- Much hard work is involved.
- You need good support.
- You need to be able to ask for help early.
- You need to be prepared to feel out of your depth.
- Many people don't see junior doctors as leaders.
- You need to be tactful.
- Think small scale.
- Good time management is essential.

What they felt they had learned is summed up by one of the trainees at the conclusion of the academic programme and highlights how leadership can and should become part of everyday practice for doctors at all levels.

As leaders, we seem to have grasped where we fit in the system; we analyse situations and understand the environment in which we work . . . I think this places us in a better position to take on leadership roles in the future. In our current role as F2s, our leadership opportunities are limited, mostly due to perceived lack of power. However, the knowledge we have now has given us insight into our future roles and how we can create momentum to drive change (F2 leader, cohort 1).

Chapter summary

This chapter has:

- provided an overview of medical leadership in the current UK NHS context;

- outlined key leadership theories and approaches with reference to clinical leadership;

- linked leadership activities with the *Medical Leadership Competency Framework*;

- provided case examples and activities to help develop leadership understanding and skills.

GOING FURTHER

Bolden, R (2004) *What is Leadership?* Exeter: University of Exeter Centre for Leadership Studies.

Dickenson, H and Ham, C (2008) *Engaging Doctors in Leadership: A Review of the Literature*. Birmingham: NHS Institute for Innovation and Improvement, University of Birmingham and Academy of Medical Royal Colleges.

McKimm, J and Phillips, K (2009) *Leadership and Management in Integrated Services*. Exeter: Learning Matters.

Stanton, E, Lemer, C and Mountford, J (2010) *Clinical Leadership: Bridging the Divide*. London: Quay Books.

Swanwick, T and McKimm, J (2011) *ABC of Clinical Leadership*. Oxford: Wiley-Blackwell.

part 5

Teaching and Research Skills

chapter 15

Learning and Teaching

Clare Morris

Achieving foundation competences

This chapter will help you begin to meet the following syllabus and competences set out in the *Foundation Programme Curriculum 2010*.

Outcome 13: Teaching and training

Outcome: demonstrates the knowledge, skills, attitudes and behaviours to undertake a teaching role.

Competences

F1

- Undertakes teaching in under- or postgraduate education in a one-to-one setting.
- Assesses students and other non-medical colleagues in training.
- Contributes to the assessment or review of students and other colleagues with whom they work.

F2

- Sets educational objectives, identifies learning needs (own and group's) and applies teaching methods appropriately.
- Demonstrates appropriate preparation for teaching.
- Undertakes small group teaching, including a presentation.
- Provides constructive feedback to others including F1 doctors.

Assessment: *Developing the clinical teacher.*

Knowledge

- Adult learning theories.
- Learner-centred approach.
- Principles of assessment.
- Principles of feedback.
- Features of an effective presentation.

It also touches upon the additional competences found for teaching in the *Compendium of Academic Competences* (UK Foundation Programme Office, 2009a), including those for small group teaching, large group teaching, bedside teaching and assessment.

Chapter overview

The General Medical Council (GMC) notes that 'teaching skills are not innate but can be learned' (GMC, 1999) and over the past decade, there has been a growing expectation that all doctors will not only be involved in teaching but also that they will be competent to teach. This expectation formally begins in the foundation years, although many medical students become involved in peer teaching before then. This chapter explores some key ideas about learning and teaching. It aims to provide you with a framework that will enable you to effectively support learning and to plan for teaching large groups, small groups and on a one-to-one basis. This chapter should be read in conjunction with Chapter 2, where some key educational terminology and principles of assessment and appraisal are introduced.

At the end of this chapter you will be able to:

- have a firm grasp of some key guiding principles to underpin your approaches to teaching in a range of settings;
- be able to adopt some strategies that will allow you to effectively prepare for a wide range of teaching encounters, including large group, small group and one-to-one teaching;
- be able to select from a range of interactive teaching and facilitation methods.

Context: the doctor as teacher

In recent years we have seen a number of moves to professionalise medical education and training. As noted above, the GMC's *The Doctor as Teacher* (1999) made explicit the need for all doctors to be engaged in supporting the development of others and to prepare themselves for this role. Generic Standards for Training (GMC, 2010e) also encompasses standards for trainers and educational supervisors who now need to be specifically selected and prepared for their roles. There has been a rapid proliferation of masters' level programmes in medical education which attract doctors across all stages of their professional careers, from foundation doctors to Directors of Medical Education. Service level commitments, shift working and working time directives have put a squeeze on opportunities to learning in and from the workplace. Teaching time is precious: strategies adopted have to effectively support learning. It is perhaps unsurprising therefore, that undergraduate and postgraduate curriculum frameworks now make explicit a range of competences for teaching, learning and assessment nor that a new workplace-based assessment tool (WPBA) *Developing the Clinical Teacher* has been introduced in the foundation years as part of the e-portfolio assessment.

Clearly, education is a vast discipline and it is not possible to cover all aspects of teaching practice nor do full justice to educational theories and perspectives in a single chapter. However, we can distil down some key principles for practice which are underpinned by sound educational thinking. The following case study provides a starting point for this process.

Case study 15.1: Enhancing the quality of clinical education

The East of England Deanery and the University of Bedfordshire have been working together to enhance the quality of medical and dental education across their region in a range of ways. In 2009 they introduced a bespoke Postgraduate Certificate (PGCert) in Medical Education, for 20 specialty trainees, selected by heads of school. These trainees are becoming involved in a range of faculty development initiatives in and across their specialty schools as part of the programme. On the last contact day of their PGCert, they were asked to think back over the programme to identify the features of 'good teaching' that they would want to share with their peers. Their responses can be organised into four key themes.

Being prepared

Being prepared means: knowing your learner(s) starting point and planning on this basis; being purposeful (having clear aims and structure); thinking about what learners will do as well as what the teacher will do during the session; ensuring relevance (to learners and learning context); creating a positive learning environment with appropriate layout and seating, basic 'comfort' needs attended to, with interruptions keep to the minimum and planning appropriately within time constraints (always keeping to time).

Using a range of strategies

This includes developing a repertoire of teaching strategies that allow interaction with large and small groups; enhanced communication skills to foster a dialogue with learners; skilled use of questioning which goes beyond testing knowledge to develop understanding, problem solving and reasoning skills and a multi-dimensional approach to teaching which draws upon a range of audio and visual resources.

Being a role model

Being a role model means displaying a positive attitude towards the practice of medicine, teaching and learning; being passionate about what you do; being approachable and affable with all learners; knowing your limitations, being open about them and seeking assistance when required; adopting a reflective and reflexive stance to your teaching and being open and responsive to feedback from learners.

Learner-centredness

Being learner-centred means shifting your thinking from teaching to learning. This means knowing your learner(s) starting points and being responsive and adaptable during teaching sessions, to ensure learners' needs are balanced with your own objectives. Being learner centred also includes:

- active listening as well as talking, giving and receiving feedback;
- setting appropriate levels of challenge while being supportive;
- engaging in an ongoing dialogue with your learner, which is mutually respectful of each others' positions and perspectives.

The case study highlights the complexity of being a 'good teacher' and the importance of thinking about learners and their learning. The features the trainees identify are underpinned by a range of thinking about adult and experiential learning which will be explored in the next section.

ACTIVITY 15.1 WHAT IS GOOD TEACHING?

- What do you see as being the key features of 'good teaching'?
- To what extent are they similar to those identified by the specialty trainees in Case study 15.1?
- To what extent are you surprised (or sceptical) about any of the identified features above?

Basic principles: keeping it real

There is a vast body of educational literature, spanning several educational schools of thought and their associated 'big thinkers'. There is no easy answer to the question 'what is the best way to teach or support learning?' Different writers on the subject will place emphasis on different aspects, although it is possible to identify some common themes.

ACTIVITY 15.2 EDUCATIONAL 'BIG THINKERS'

The underpinning principles identified in this chapter draw on the work of John Dewey (1897), Malcolm Knowles (1983), David Kolb (1984), Jean Lave and Etienne Wenger (1991). A summary and critique of their contributions can be found on the 'encyclopaedia of informal education website' (Infed) at **www.infed.org**. Visit the website and take some time to familiarise yourself with their ideas about learning.

- What do they seem to have in common?
- What stands out as being particularly important about their contribution?
- Which of these 'thinkers' particularly appeals to you and why?

Drawing upon a range of educational thinking, it is possible to identify some shared principles that are useful in helping to critique different approaches to teaching as well as guide us in our own teaching practices. These are summed up in the simple mnemonic (REAL), illustrated in Figure 15.1.

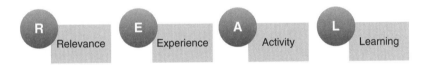

Figure 15.1 REAL learning

Relevance

The trainees in our case study emphasised the importance of knowing and responding to your learners' starting points and ensuring that teaching was relevant to their needs. Whilst the need to pass examinations is often a driving force in medical education, we need to be mindful that the primary goal is to improve patient care. We can do this by ensuring that our teaching is always strongly connected to medical practice. In 1897 John Dewey, a philosopher and radical reformer of education, laid out his pedagogic creed. His critique of the school system at the time is remarkably similar to criticisms levied at some forms of professional education today.

> I believe that education, therefore, is a process of living and not a preparation for future living. . . . I believe that much of present education fails because it neglects this fundamental principle of the school as a form of community life. It conceives the school as a place where certain information is to be given, where certain lessons are to be learned, or where certain habits are to be formed. The value of

these is conceived as lying largely in the remote future; the child must do these things for the sake of something else he is to do; they are mere preparation. As a result they do not become a part of the life experience of the child and so are not truly educative.

(Dewey, 1897)

If we relate Dewey's ideas to medical education, we need to consider how all stages of training are truly educative, enabling students and trainees to be as actively engaged in medical practice as it is safe for them to be so. This is easy to translate into clinical teaching practices, where students are able to become engaged in some aspects of patient care (for example, taking histories, explaining procedures, performing simple procedural skills, examining patients, etc.). In more formal settings it is about bringing teaching to life with real case examples and the use of clinical material. Rather than seeing teaching as a chance to tell students everything you know, try seeing it as an opportunity to help them rehearse the types of thinking skills that are vital in medical education such as clinical reasoning, diagnostic skills or analysing and interpreting clinical data. Dewey was very clear about the importance of problem solving and that teachers should not impose certain ideas, rather both learners and teachers should be part of a learning community where teachers select experiences that help learners develop their thinking.

Experience

The value of drawing on experience therefore, extends from the need to ensure relevance. If medical education is to be relevant to medical practice, both teacher and learner need to engage with a wide range of experiences of medical practice. For the teacher, this means bringing teaching to life by drawing upon exemplars, using story telling and narrative to illustrate principles and practices. It means bringing the clinical into the classroom, using authentic materials and data. One rule of thumb when planning any type of teaching is to identify what it is that you can offer that a textbook can't – which is, of course, the lived experience of being a doctor. But it also means considering how your learners engage with their experiences of being in medical workplaces and observing and engaging with medical practice. You need to think about how you can help them draw upon and make sense of these experiences in a range of ways. You will also need to think about the types of experiences you offer them and how to make the best use of them. Knowles' writing on adult learning (andragogy) is often cited and emphasises the fact that life experience is a rich reservoir for learning which should be built upon (Knowles, 1983). Links can be seen with Kolb's (1984) model of experiential learning. Whilst it is possible to criticise the model for the lack of attention paid to the role of the teacher in guiding learners towards and through appropriate learning experiences, it does draw attention to potentially useful ways of fostering experiential learning.

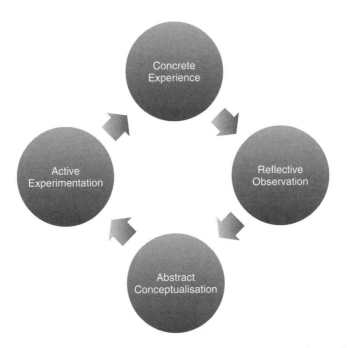

Figure 15.2 Representation of Kolb's cycle of experiential learning (after Kolb, 1984)

So, let us apply this model to a practical example. You wish to help your students develop their skills in taking a history from a confused patient. You ask them to work in pairs, each taking a short history from a patient on the ward, carefully observing each other (concrete experience). In the reflective observation stage you might ask them to debrief together, identifying difficulties encountered and differences of approach and related outcomes (reflective observation). You might then meet with them and help them identify what might be behind the difficulties encountered (i.e. the cognitive and behavioural manifestations of confusion and how this impacts on usual history taking practices). You might also encourage them to think about ways round the problems they encountered, encouraging them to think of differences in approach (abstract conceptualisation). Finally, you might invite them to try out some of their proposed strategies and see how they work (active experimentation). This in turn takes you back to the experience stage. Whilst there is a tendency to start with the concrete experience, you could start any where in the cycle; for example, with a conversation about why it is challenging to take a history from a confused patient (abstract conceptualisation).

ACTIVITY 15.3 APPLYING KOLB'S MODEL

Imagine you were asked to help some medical students learn how to interpret ECGs. How might you use Kolb's model as a guide to planning? Identify two different ways to do this, with two different starting points in the model.

Activity

We have already started thinking about the ways in which you might encourage learners to be actively engaged in learning experiences – be it encouraging them to think things through for themselves, or to try out new skills. What has yet to be emphasised is the importance of the shared experience of learning; in other words, the interactions between teachers and learners and between learners themselves. Dewey articulates this as follows:

> I believe that the active side precedes the passive in the development of the child nature; . . . I believe that the neglect of this principle is the cause of a large part of the waste of time and strength in school work. The child is thrown into a passive, receptive or absorbing attitude.
>
> (Dewey, 1897, pp77–80)

Dewey's thinking can be traced in the work of many other educational thinkers within the constructivist school of thought. They argue that learning arises from an interaction between ideas and experiences, these experiences taking place in a social world. Whilst there is value in didactic teaching in some circumstances, it is dangerous to assume that there is a causal relationship between teaching and learning! Students need to test out new ideas, hold them up to past experience, consider how they relate to what others might say (other teachers, peers, a recently read article or book chapter, or a patient they saw in clinic) and decide (however unconsciously) whether to accept or reject the new ideas and modify their thinking. This may happen outside the classroom – but can happen more powerfully if opportunities for this type of activity are built into learning sessions. When planning learning, it is important to plan not only what you will do but also what students will do and achieve.

Learning

The trainees in the case study highlight the importance of learner centredness, a phrase that appears in the Foundation Programme documentation. Learning is an important part of the guiding mnemonic for two reasons: being learner-centred and being part of a learning community.

Being learner-centred means shifting your attention from teaching to learning and making sure your input is directed towards learners needs. This has been explored in relation to the REA aspects of the REAL mnemonic above. Being part of a learning community (or 'community of practice' as Lave and Wenger (1991) might suggest) means extending the thinking beyond learning as something that is an individual pursuit that happens as a result of engagements between teacher and learner. Medicine takes place in diverse communities, with successful patient outcomes being dependent upon effective working relationships between all community members, including patients and their carers. No matter how brilliant the surgeon in a team, she or he cannot function without other members of the surgical team, including nurses, ODPs, anaesthetists, theatre managers, administrative staff organising waiting lists, theatre porters and so on. Students may learn with you and from you, but they can also learn with other members of the team and from patients themselves. Approaches to teaching that maximise learning within communities are vitally important.

Being prepared

The REAL mnemonic provides a helpful starting point for all types of teaching; in other words, you need to ask yourself 'how can I make it REAL?' Some types of teaching naturally tap into these key guiding principles. Clinical teaching may feel opportunistic and relatively unstructured, but it is easy to make it relevant, draw on experience, actively involve learners and the wider learning community. Traditional didactic lectures may be more of a challenge.

ACTIVITY 15.4 KEEPING IT REAL

Think about a typical lecture, small group tutorial and bedside teaching session. For each session consider the extent to which it is possible to ensure they are 'REAL'. What steps could you take to ensure they were as 'REAL' as possible?

Learning needs analysis

A starting point for all preparation has to be a learning needs analysis, that is, establishing your learner(s) starting point(s) and plan accordingly (McKimm and Swanwick, 2010) and see also Table 15.1.

Table 15.1 Examples of ways to establish learning needs

Lectures	Small Group Work	One-to-One Teaching
Explore knowledge base: quiz at start of lecture to identify any common gaps in knowledge	Explore knowledge base: quiz or ask groups of three to make a flip chart poster of top ten facts about the topic	Socratic type questions to explore knowledge base (see below)
Explore knowledge application/ use: data interpretation activity (reading ECG/X-ray, identifying visible signs/symptoms) to identify common gaps in understanding	Explore knowledge use/application: use paper cases or scenarios and ask students to identify three aspects they would find most challenging	Counselling type questions to explore attitudes/feelings (see below)
Explore attitudes: e.g. stand up/ put your hand up if very confident about this aspect, quite confident, low confidence, no confidence, etc.	Explore attitudes: use line ups. Draw an imaginary likert scale on the floor with each end representing an extreme point (high/low confidence, high/low belief) and ask students to arrange themselves on it in response	'Diagnostic assessment', e.g. use of (or review of) workplace based assessment tools

to statements (The NHS should not treat smokers . . .)

Invite questions: start lecture with overview and then ask students to write any burning questions on a sticky note and pass to end of row to collect. Review these while they undertake a quick data interpretation task or similar	Explore starting positions: ask students to explain a condition in lay terms (as if to a patient) to establish starting assumptions. Challenge them to re-explain the condition as if to a supervising consultant at the end of the session.	Observed practice (with patients or in simulation if obvious patient safety risk)

Learning outcomes

Having established learning needs, the next stage is to agree learning outcomes. This process can range from a very informal on-the-spot goal setting ('ok, so with the next patient, your goal is to take the history demonstrating much more active listening this time') to a formal process of crafting outcomes which will be formally assessed in an end of unit examination, for example. For each the principles are the same – they must indicate to the learner exactly what is required in terms of demonstrable knowledge, skills or attitudes, at the end of a period of learning. Bloom's taxonomy can be used to ensure your outcomes have an appropriate level of cognitive challenge: you want to be moving your learners from factual recall (knowledge) to much higher levels of thought (analysis, synthesis and application). Table 15.2 illustrates this point, providing some guiding verbs and an exemplar of learning outcomes for the topic 'workplace-based assessments'.

ACTIVITY 15.5 IDENTIFYING LEARNING OUTCOMES

Imagine you had been asked to teach some final year medical students for an hour about the use and interpretation of ECGs.

- Can you identify a learning outcome for each of the six levels?
- What methods might you use to assess whether they had achieved your outcomes?

Structure

Whatever the type of teaching undertaken, structure is important. This starts with identifying learning needs and outcomes, whilst providing a clear context for what is about to follow. The main 'body' of the teaching session should also include explicit signposting ('we have looked at this, now lets look at that'). In the final section of any

Table 15.2 Linking learning outcomes to cognitive levels (after Bloom, 1956).

Evaluation

- e.g. criticise, appraise, justify, argue, debate, judge
- *Judge the fitness for purpose of WPBA tools as a way to identify and support the development of underperforming trainees*

Synthesis

- e.g. hypothesise, formulate, propose, predict,
- *Formulate a case against the summative use of WPBA*

Analysis

- e.g. analyse, investigate, differentiate
- *Differentiate between the uses of Mini-CEX, DOPS and CbD*

Application

- e.g. solve, report, modify, classify, categorise
- *categorise the listed assessment tools on the basis of their use being formative, summative or both*

Comprehension

- e.g. describe, outline, summarise, explain
- *explain how multi-source feedback works*

Knowledge

- e.g. list, define, identify, label, state
- *Name the five WPBA used in the foundation years*

session, you should also allow time to summarise, check understanding and identify next steps. The AMEE (Association for Medical Education in Europe) Guide on Refreshing Lecturing (Brown and Manogue, 2001) provides an excellent overview of different ways to structure medical lectures to develop student understanding. For example, the problem-orientated lecture starts by posing a clinical problem (e.g. using a paper case to explore most likely reasons for a patient's presenting signs and symptoms) that contrasts with more classical lectures which tend to follow a textbook format. The problem-orientated lecture is more likely to allow you to embrace the REAL principle, and to enable you to offer students something a text book can't.

Use a range of strategies

Interaction and facilitation

There is a common misconception that interactive teaching strategies are only possible with small groups or in one-to-one teaching. This may be because novice teachers think purely in terms of interactions between teacher and learners (typically in the form of Question and Answer sessions). Table 15.3 illustrates four different types of interaction that may be used in a range of teaching formats.

Table 15.3 Ideas for different types of 'interactions'

Own ideas	*Data*
• Write down three things you have learned and one unanswered question you will follow up • Take a couple of minutes to write down what you would do next if you had taken this history • Consider what might be your own strengths and development needs in relation to this patient encounter • Think back to the last WPBA and identify the most pressing development need	• The legend for the Y axis is missing on this graph . . . what might it be (and why) • What is the most likely explanation for this ECG trace? • Comment as you can on this patient's presentation (photo images) • Here are the investigation results for Mr X. What further investigation might you wish to undertake . . . justify your choice
Each other	*The teacher*
• Now you have completed the quiz, compare your answers with the person beside you • Talk to those around you and find out if anyone has seen a patient with this condition and what they would add to what I have said so far • Do a straw poll in your group (along your row) to find out the most popular diagnosis on the basis of this case information • Talk to those around you and establish three reasons why it may be difficult to take a history from . . . (e.g. the parents of a very sick child)	• Prepare 'gapped handouts' that have to be completed during the session • Agree when you are willing to take questions – use questions on sticky notes if you prefer to take them at the end • Whole group questioning (hands up if you think the answer is a, b or c) • Whole group attitude scanning – stand up now if you agree with this statement (then disagree, are neutral etc.) • Ask each row/group to come up with a really good question to ask you half way through the teaching session

A number of helpful resources are available to help you think of creative ways to engage learners including e-learning resources designed for clinical teachers as well as downloadable toolkits for facilitators. It is worth spending some time looking at these, as well as to be open to picking up tips from your own teachers. See the end of this chapter for links.

Questions

Questioning can be a very powerful teaching method. We have looked at how it can form the basis of a learning needs analysis and you will all have experienced it as a method of establishing your knowledge base. But questioning can also be used to extend and develop thinking and reasoning in a range of ways. You may already have got a sense of this in Activity 15.5 when you thought about developing a range of learning outcomes on a particular topic: each of these could be turned into a question to invite your learners to think aloud.

The way in which you ask questions is important. Rather than bombarding or interrogating, use questions to invite thought as part of a developmental conversation with your learners.

ACTIVITY 15.6 QUESTIONING TECHNIQUES

Imagine you are doing some clinical teaching about Mr Jones who is 45 and has presented with a possible myocardial infarction. Think of a different question about this patient, for each of the following learners:

- A first-year medical student on an early patient experience placement.
- A third-year medical student at the start of a 10-week medical attachment.
- A third-year medical student at the end of a 10-week medical attachment.
- A FY1 doctor at the start of the year.
- A FY1 doctor at the end of the year.

Review your questions now. How many started with the word 'what'? Whilst 'what' questions are good for checking knowledge, they may not develop thinking at all levels (encouraging application, synthesis – remember Blooms cognitive levels above). Think again and see if you can identify appropriate questions starting with 'why', 'how', 'who', 'when', etc.

You may find it helpful to distinguish between different approaches to questioning. For example, a 'Socratic' approach aims to help learners examine their ideas in a critical way, both eliciting and extending their understanding of issues. Socratic questions aim to help learners clarify concepts, explore assumptions, articulate their reasoning and evidence base, consider a range of viewpoints or perspectives on an issue and examine implications of a position. This method is often employed in teaching law and medicine, with bedside teaching providing some wonderful examples. The 'heuristic' approach on the other hand aims to promote discovery, using questions to stimulate learners' curiosity and interest in topics through problem-solving and trial and error. Problem-based learning is based on this principle, where problems act as triggers for learners to identify the ways in which they might develop a greater understanding of the issues arising. A 'counselling' approach will aim to explore emotional dimensions of learning and practice and may be particularly important if you have a learner who seems reluctant to engage, or seems 'stuck' in their thinking.

To illustrate, imagine you had been asked to teach a medical student about communication problems following stroke. A Socratic line of questioning might be 'so you have told me the two types of problems are dysarthria and dysphasia, what do you see as the key distinctions between them?' or 'given this patient has cerebelar damage, can you explain to me why they are more likely to be dysarthric than dysphasic?' A heuristic line of questioning might be 'what different types of problems have you faced when talking to patients who have communication problems following a stroke? Who in the team might be best placed to help you understand these differences and how to adapt your communication skills when talking to these patients?' A counselling line of questioning might be 'Can you think about a situation where you have had difficulty making yourself understood – how did it feel? What helped? Can you draw parallels with dysphasic patients? What might help you communicate with them more effectively?"

ACTIVITY 15.7

You will find some excellent starting points for Socratic questioning on the Changing Minds website at: **http://changingminds.org/techniques/questioning/socratic_questions.htm**

Go back to the Mr Jones teaching scenario in Activity 15.6 and see if you can identify a range of Socratic type questions to develop your learners' thinking.

Feedback

Chapter 2 introduced the value of feedback and the role it plays in workplace-based assessment, appraisal and supervision. Feedback is described as a 'developmental conversation', with the emphasis being on a two-way dialogue which has the developmental needs of the learner in mind. Effective feedback needs to feed-forward too, identifying short and longer terms goals for improvement, linked to clear action planning and including review periods. One way to think about feedback is that it rehearses the skills necessary to critically appraise your own performance. Self-appraisal is at the heart of safe, autonomous practice and enables learners to recognise the limits of their abilities and when to seek advice or assistance. All learners have the right to expect regular, developmental feedback conversations: even the most able trainee should be challenged to develop further.

There are a number of models for giving feedback, but there are no set rules. Some general principles for learner-centred feedback are provided below, which focus on context, dialogue, development and action.

- Context: be mindful of time, place and readiness of learner.

- Dialogue: this should be a two-way process, with the learner leading (in order to rehearse skills).

- Development: as well as looking back, you must look forward, identifying the learning arising from the experience.

- Action: make sure you identify immediate goals for development, link those to forthcoming learning opportunities and consider the support your learner may need to achieve these.

> ### What's the evidence? Improving self-assessment through feedback
>
> A systematic review of the effectiveness of self-assessment in identifying learning needs was unable to identify a robust evidence base to answer their intended questions. However, the team notes:
>
> > there was some evidence that the accuracy of self-assessment can be enhanced by feedback, particularly video and verbal, and by providing explicit assessment criteria and benchmarking guidance. There was also some evidence that the least competent are also the least able to self-assess accurately.
> >
> > (Colthart et al., 2007, p9)

Developing the clinical teacher

The new WPBA tool (*Developing the Clinical Teacher*) found in the foundation e-portfolio provides a helpful way to conclude this chapter. Your development as a clinical teacher is something that starts in medical school but will continue throughout your medical career. This chapter has introduced you to some of the thinking underpinning a learner-centred approach to medical education as well some strategies to try out in a range of teaching encounters. The going further section below points you to some free online resources available for clinical teachers. There are increasing opportunities to develop as a clinical teacher with information available on short courses and workshops in faculty development on the websites of your local deaneries and medical schools as well as relevant medical royal colleges. You may also wish to consider undertaking a master's level award in medical or clinical education as you move into the training grades.

> ### Chapter summary
>
> - All doctors have a responsibility to teach and need to invest time in developing the skills to do so.
>
> - By drawing upon the 'REAL' principles (relevance, experience, activity and learning) teaching becomes increasingly learner-centred.
>
> - Purposeful preparation is key.
>
> - A range of strategies can be used to engage your learners and develop their thinking.

GOING FURTHER

The London Deanery Faculty Development Unit offer free e-learning modules at **www.faculty.londondeanery.ac.uk/e-learning**. You will find useful resources on facilitating learning in the workplace, lecturing, small group teaching and feedback.

This website also provides helpful links to a range of other educational resources. You can access a link to download a Facilitators Toolkit produced by the NHS Institute for Innovation and Improvement as well as a series of articles under the heading 'Clinical Teaching Made Easy' which appeared in the *British Journal for Hospital Medicine*. These are available at: **www.faculty.londondeanery. ac.uk/other-resources** and as a book *Clinical Teaching Made Easy*, published by Quay Books.

Acknowledgements

Thank you to the trainees completing the PGCert in Medical Education at the University of Bedforshire who generously shared their views on 'good teaching' for the case study in this chapter.

chapter 16

Research Skills

Brian D. Nicholson

Achieving foundation competences

This chapter will help you to begin to meet the following requirements of the *Foundation Programme Curriculum* (2010).

12.2 Research, evidence, guidelines and care protocols
Outcome: demonstrates the knowledge, skills, attitudes and behaviours to use evidence and guidelines that will improve patient care.

Competences
F1 and F2

- Finds and interprets evidence relating to clinical questions.
- Supports patients in interpreting evidence.
- Appraises recent research, and discusses findings with colleagues to advocate specific action.

Assessment MSF, CBD and mini-CEX.

Knowledge

- Evidence based medicine (EBM).
- Guidelines and protocols.
- Limitations of the existing evidence base.
- Advantages and limitations of guidelines and protocols.
- Methods of determining best practice.

The chapter will also introduce you to the Research Outcomes set out in the *Compendium of Academic Competencies* published by the UK Foundation Programme Office (UKFPO, 2009)

The 13 core outcomes are broken down into the following three groupings:

Research planning

- Question formulation.
- Critically appraise a topic.

- Systematically review a topic.
- Write a research proposal.
- Write an application for funding.
- Write an application for ethics approval.

Conduct of research

- Carry out a lab-based experiment, analyse the results and write a report.
- Carry out a research study involving human volunteers or NHS patients.
- Carry out a population-based study, analyse the results and write a report.
- Take informed consent for a research project.

Dissemination

- Write up a study for publication in a peer-reviewed journal.
- Present the results as a poster presentation.
- Present the results as an oral presentation.

Chapter overview

By conducting research, we aim to generate new evidence to add to the existing literature base for our topic of choice. As a foundation doctor you will be asked to conduct clinical audit and regularly discuss the literature with your colleagues. As an academic foundation doctor you will be expected to devise and conduct your own research project.

After reading this chapter you will be prepared to:

- understand evidence-based medicine;
- generate precise research questions;
- search and understand the literature;
- critically appraise the evidence;
- select the correct study design;
- conduct your research paying attention to safety, confidentiality, and ethics;
- disseminate your results.

Generating hypotheses and questions

Teachings by Karl Popper (1902–94), eminent professor of philosophy at London School of Economics, led to the hypothetico-deductive approach to scientific research that now underpins the generation of scientific evidence and the formation of clinical reasoning. Using the hypothetico-deductive method, the clinician uses information from history and examination to generate tentative hypotheses.

Hypotheses are then followed by the collection and interpretation of further patient data, such as blood tests and imaging. Continued hypothesis creation and evaluation takes place as examination and management evolves. Our various hypotheses are confirmed or disproved until a diagnosis is made.

Through his work on falsifiability, Professor Popper, furthering earlier work by William Whewell (1794–1866), proposed the 'null hypothesis', realising it was not always possible to prove a hypothesis, but more helpful to follow the pursuit of disproving or falsifying hypotheses (Popper, 1935). A null hypothesis states that the results are nothing more than chance; for example, 'salbutamol inhalers provide no benefit in mild intermittent asthma'. We rarely believe our null hypothesis, but from this starting point we can carefully construct a study to generate evidence relevant to our clinical suspicions.

The phrase 'evidence-based medicine' (EBM) was coined by Gordon Guyatt (b. 1953), Professor of Clinical Epidemiology and Biostatistics at McMaster University, who challenged clinicians to use more epidemiological evidence when making clinical decisions (Guyatt, 1992).

In a seminal 1996 *British Medical Journal* (BMJ) editorial, Professor David Sackett and colleagues of the then NHS Research and Development Centre for Evidence Based Medicine defined EBM as 'the conscientious, explicit, and judicious use of the current best evidence in making decisions about the care of individual patients'. Clinically relevant evidence came 'sometimes from basic science, but especially from patient-centred clinical research into the accuracy of diagnostic tests, the power of prognostic markers, and the efficacy & safety of interventions' (Sackett et al., 1996).

Today, we use a later definition from Sackett: 'Evidence based medicine is the integration of best research evidence, with clinical expertise and patient values, to achieve the best possible management' (Straus et al., 2010).

So, in designing a research project we must first generate a hypothesis to test, or a clinical question to answer. A widely used method for question generation is the PICO formula.

The PICO formula

It is widely accepted that a flawed research question will result in the generation of irrelevant answers. The PICO formula is a tool adopted by leaders in the world of EBM for precise, specific question building. Time spent at this stage will inevitably save time and effort gathering and analysing unnecessary or inappropriate data. PICO can also be used as a tool to help clarify study design when reading through the evidence.

PICO (Patient or Problem, Intervention or Exposure, Comparison, Outcome) acknowledges that a well-built clinical question contains four key elements:

- *Population/Problem*: How you would describe or define your patient group?

- *Intervention (or Exposure)*: Describe the intervention you are studying (this could be a cause, prognostic factor, or treatment).

- *Comparison (if necessary)*: Decide what the main comparative group will be (another treatment, the standard alternative therapy, no therapy, a placebo).

- *Outcome*: What outcome are you interested in?

If you are specific and precise during the PICO process you may distil your research question down to only a small number of words. For example, using five-year survival data, your supervisor asks you to investigate whether a newly developed drug A is more effective than older drug B at treating patients with cancer of the stomach:

P: Stomach cancer. *I*: Drug A. *C*: Drug B. *O*: Improved five-year survival. *Question*: In stomach cancer, does drug A, compared to drug B, improve five-year survival?

Through breaking the process down in this way we also simplify the next step of the research process, searching the literature.

Understanding the literature

In EBM it is vital not only to read papers, but also to read the correct papers at the right time. The huge volume of medical literature out there is demonstrated by the fact that there are hundreds of journals dedicated to summarising the key research findings of others. To make sense of it all you must first be aware of how to success-fully navigate through the literature and, second, of how the evidence fits together.

Searching the literature

There are many varied search engines and databases available online. Nothing beats the advice of your local librarian and, to maximise your time spent trawling through the world's medical literature, most university libraries will run training sessions of the most relevant up-to-date literature search skills and tools. Some places to start include:

- PubMED (pubmed.com): indexing over 20 million citations going back to 1865 and maintained by The United States National Library of Medicine (NLM); for primary research, PubMED is still the most comprehensive.

- NHS Evidence (evidence.nhs.uk): launched April 2009, free to access, and free article download with your NHS Athens password. This is an excellent and growing resource which is part of the UK health policy push towards improved access to high-quality evidence collating varied evidence from sources including National Institute for Health and Clinical Excellence guidelines, the Medical Royal Colleges' publications, medical charities' reports and research, the Cochrane sys-tematic review database, Clinical Knowledge Summaries, and primary research.

- Clinical Evidence (clinicalevidence.bmj.com) and Health Information Resources (library.nhs.uk) are both great sites with excellent links to other evidence-based resources.

- TRIP Database (tripdatabase.com): innovative, committed to evidence-based medicine, joining is free, and they collate your search results by evidence type including up-to-date clinical guidelines (NB: the forward-thinking developing world feature).

- Google Scholar: research suggests that Google Scholar is catching up with other specialist databases, but at present lacks precision when compared for example to PubMED. One to watch.

Search tips

Starting with your PICO output, use the MeSH function (Medical Sub-Headings, **www.ncbi.nlm.nih.gov/mesh**) to identify related search terms from within the complex matrix of medical terminology used to index PubMED.

When searching use the asterisk '*' which traditionally stems a search term so you may search for variant endings. For example 'diabet*' will search for diabetes, diabetic, diabetogenic, etc. The hash symbol '#' replaces definite but variable characters: summari#e where '#' could be 's' or 'z'. The question mark '?' indicates there may or may not be a character in the specified location: an?esthetics' where '?' could resemble a 'blank' or an 'a', or in 'colo?r' where ? could resemble a 'blank' or 'u', taking into consideration common international spelling variations.

Publication bias

Beware, publication bias comes in various guises, but in essence is the fact that studies with negative findings tend not to get published as often as positive ones. It can be summarised as follows, with statistically significant 'positive' results being more likely to be:

- published (publication bias);

- published rapidly (time lag bias);

- published in English (language bias);

- published more than once (multiple publication bias);

- and cited by others (citation bias).

This information is taken from the Cochrane collaborations excellent open-learning module on publication bias, from their systematic review and meta-analysis teaching found at (**www.cochrane-net.org/openlearning/HTML/mod15.htm**).

For completeness and to help avoid publication bias, you should take care to include studies reported in non-English-speaking journals. Many journals have translations available, and the internet has many translation sites to help you. You should also include unpublished evidence and grey literature within your search. This can come, for example, from personal contact with prominent authors or research institutions in your field of study, by asking for additional data, unpublished reports, or personal correspondence documenting new developments, and up-to-date opinion.

The hierarchy of evidence

You should be aware of the traditional 'hierarchy of evidence' (Figure 16.1), or the phrase 'level of evidence' used to demonstrate how reliable a study is by starting with the most robust at the top (for more information on these study types see the methodology section).

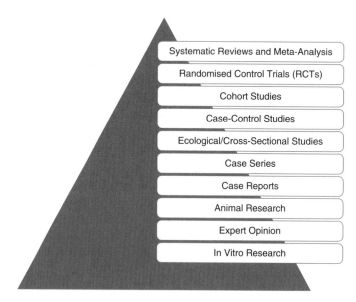

Figure 16.1 The hierarchy of evidence

Grading the literature: producing clinical guidelines

Grading schemes have existed for over 25 years to generate appropriate clinical guidance from the wide range of available evidence. A clinical guideline is a systematically developed statement based on graded evidence to assist practitioner decisions about appropriate healthcare for specific clinical circumstances. The resultant 'levels of evidence' approach is now commonplace in the UK demonstrated by NICE (National Institute for Health and Clinical Excellence) guidelines.

Since 1999 the Scottish Intercollegiate Guideline Network (SIGN) have been at the forefront of producing evidence-based clinical guidelines, basing their judgement entirely on study design. Tables 16.1 and 16.2 show how SIGN turns the levels of evidence into evidence grades for use in clinical guidelines. A complete guide to clinical guideline development can be found at **www.sign.ac.uk/guidelines/fulltext/50/ index.html**.

Table 16.1 Levels of evidence

Level 1	**Evidence from meta-analysis, systematic reviews of RCTS, and RCTS**
1++	Very low risk of bias
1+	Low risk of bias
1–	High risk of bias
Level 2	**Evidence from case-control studies or cohort studies, including sytematic reviews of case-control studies and cohort studies**
2++	Very low risk of bias, confounding or chance
	High probability the relationship is causal
2+	Low risk of bias, confounding or chance
	Moderate probability the relationship is causal
2–	High risk of bias, confounding or chance
	Significant risk that the relationship is not causal
Level 3	**Evidence from non-analytic studies (case reports, case series)**
Level 4	**Expert opinion**

Table 16.2 Grading (A, B, C, D, good practice points) of evidence

A	At least *one 1++ study* directly applicable to the target population demonstrating overall consistency of results *or,* A *body of 1+ studies* directly applicable to the target population demonstrating overall consistency of results.
B	A *body of 2+ studies* directly applicable to the target population with overall consistency of results *or,* *Extrapolated evidence from 1++ or 1+*
C	A *body of 2+ studies* directly applicable to the target population with overall consistency of results *or,* *Extrapolated evidence from 2++*
D	*Level 3 or 4 evidence or,* *Extrapolated evidence from 2+*

Good practice points: based on the experience of the guideline development group

Grading of Recommendations Assessment, Development and Evaluation (GRADE)

In recent years GRADE has emerged through international collaboration by a team led by Professor Guyatt at McMaster University. GRADE aims to be a uniform, transparent system with which all clinicians, policy-makers and patients can become familiar. GRADE uses information in addition to the study methodology, such as risk/benefit analysis, and economic analysis. GRADE has been developed with, and taken up by, many of the world's leading health agencies such as the World Health Organisation (WHO), *British Medical Journal* (BMJ), and SIGN, as a uniform approach to recommendation generation (**www.gradeworkinggroup.org**).

Clinical audit

Whilst many tend not to be published, clinical audit remains the process by which we regularly and systematically review whether EBM is practised in the clinical setting. You will be aware of the audit cycle from your undergraduate days. The major differences between research and audit are shown in Table 16.3.

Table 16.3 Differences between research and audit

Audit	Research
Asks are we doing what we are supposed to be doing?	Asks what are we meant to be doing?
Aims to improve the quality of care	Aims to establish best practice
Is specific to a particular setting	Can be generalised to other settings
Aims to improve services	Aims to improve knowledge
Is led by service providers	Is led by researchers
Is based on practice	Is based on theory
Never involves randomly allocating patients to different treatment groups	May involve the random allocation of patients to different treatment groups
Never involves a completely new treatment	May involve a completely new treatment
Deals with clinical significance	Deals with statistical significance

Source: Cooper et al., 2006, reproduced with permission

ACTIVITY 16.1 SEARCH THE LITERATURE

Using the PICO approach, first generate a research questions in an area you are interested. Using your PICO question, search the literature using the resources provided. When searching, try to identify a range of study types as demonstrated in the hierarchy of research. Save them to refer back to later.

Critical appraisal

Publication in a peer-reviewed journal does not necessarily guarantee research quality. Critical appraisal provides us with a discipline to rigorously and systematically deconstruct the evidence in front of us, to assess its strengths and weaknesses, and so decide how useful it is in decision-making. The ability to critically appraise a paper also puts us in good stead to later design a useful piece of research of our own.

Many authors start by mentioning the familiar IMRAD (Introduction, Methods, Results, Discussion) format for papers. The vast majority of critical appraisal is done within the methods section of a paper.

How to critically appraise

The Centre for Evidence Based Medicine at Oxford University (**www.cebm.net**) hosts a vast up-to-date resource dedicated to the teaching and practice of evidence-based medicine. If you navigate to the 'critical appraisal' section of the 'tools for evidence-based medicine' section, you can find critical appraisal templates, calculators, and even software to guide you through critical appraisal for the different study types.

Critical appraisal is a skill. It takes time and practice to become proficient and confident. A paper that may take your professor a few minutes to deconstruct will take a beginner hours. There are many elements of a paper to become comfortable with: the terminology, relevance of study design, population size, appropriately used statistics, etc. For this reason many aides to critical appraisal have been developed.

The Graphic Approach to Epidemiology (GATE)

The GATE frame was developed by Rod Jackson, Professor of Clinical Epidemiology at the University of Auckland. GATE was developed to provide a simple unified theoretical framework for teaching and practising critical appraisal of all clinical epidemiological studies. GATE is based around a simple picture – the GATE frame – incorporating a triangle, a circle, a square and two arrows that graphically represent all epidemiological studies; whether they are randomised (trials) or non-randomised, longitudinal or cross-sectional. For a selection of resources providing more information on the GATE frame and on the related Critical Appraisal Topics (CATS), visit **www.epiq.co.nz**.

Standard Reporting Guidelines (SRGs)

In recent years there has been a move towards various SRGs. These are a minimum number of sets of requirements deemed necessary by expert consensus to ensure clear and transparent reporting of what was done and what was found during the research process. Designed to address issues that might introduce bias or confounding and increase reliability, SRGs are fast becoming the 'industry-standard' taken on board by high-impact journals such as *The Lancet, New England Journal of Medicine* (NEJM), *Journal of the American Medical Association* (JAMA), and the *BMJ*.

Through the use of flowchart templates, and tick-box checklists, SRGs are useful to us not only when critically appraising others, but when designing and writing up our own research. Case study 16.1 goes into more detail showing two examples of SRGs for RCTs, and systematic reviews, followed by links to other SRGs and resources.

The Enhancing the QUAlity and Transparency Of health Research network (EQUATOR) has a comprehensive list of reporting guidelines at **www.equator-net-work.org/resource-centre/library-of-health-research-reporting**. EQUATOR aims to become 'the recognised global centre providing resources, education and training relating to the reporting of health research and use of reporting guidelines'.

Case study 16.1: The rise of standard reporting guidelines

Consolidated Standards of Reporting Trials (CONSORT)

Since 1993, key members of the world's leading medical journals, universities, and academics have worked together on what is now called CONSORT (consort-statement.org). Last updated in 2010, the CONSORT statement is an 'evidence-based, minimum set of recommendations for reporting RCTs. It offers a standard way for authors to prepare reports of trial findings, facilitating their complete and transparent reporting and aiding their critical appraisal and interpretation'. What the statement boils down to is a 25-item tick-box checklist focusing on how the trial was designed, analysed, and interpreted, and a flow diagram to help display the progress of all participants through the trial. This is the gold standard for reporting RCTs and the statement, checklist, and flow-diagram templates can be downloaded free from the CONSORT website.

However, EBM is a fast-evolving speciality, and at the time of writing the Standard Protocol Items for Randomized Trials (SPIRIT), a new improved 33-item checklist to ensure that RCTs also include a minimum set of core scientific, ethical, and organisational considerations, was close to launch, most likely to replace CONSORT (**www.thelancet.com/journals/lancet/article/PIIS0140673610605235/fulltext?rss=yes**).

Preferred Reporting Items of Systematic reviews and Meta-Analyses (PRISMA)

Formerly QUality Of Reporting Of Meta-analyses (QUORUM), PRISMA is the CONSORT of Systematic Reviews and Meta-Analyses (**www.prisma-statement.org**). PRISMA is an evolving document including a 27-item checklist and a four-stage flow diagram developed by an international team led by Dr David Moher of the Ottawa Hospital Research Institute (OHRI) to improve reporting and conduct in systematic reviews.

Other SRGs include: STrengthening the Reporting of OBservational studies in Epidemiology (STROBE) (**www.strobe-statement.org**) and STAndards for the Reporting of Diagnostic accuracy studies (STARD) (**www.stard-statement.org**).

ACTIVITY 16.2 APPRAISE THE LITERATURE

Using the appropriate SRG from the Web, critically appraise one of the studies retrieved during Activity 16.1. Take time to work through the checklist and flow diagram. When finished, try to write a 250-word summary of your findings.

Study design

We have touched on the main study types through discussing grading of the evidence. A clear knowledge of the study types available will help you to choose the correct methodology to answer your clinical question precisely. Figure 16.2 shows the organisation of study types.

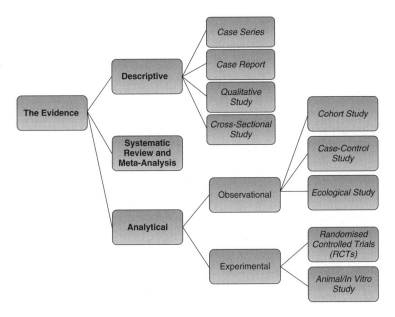

Figure 16.2 Overview and organisation of study types

Case Series/Report: an in-depth documentation and discussion surrounding a series of similar cases/or one interesting case. Often used to document an unusual or interesting disease process, to explore new areas for investigation, or report unexpected side effects.

Qualitative Study: qualitative research seeks to understand and interpret personal experience and explain social phenomena such as why people do not adhere to a treatment regimen or why a certain healthcare intervention is successful. It uses many methods of data collection, including observation, case study, interviews, focus groups, and numerous approaches to data analysis ranging from the quasi-statistical to the intuitive and inductive (Hutson and Rowan, 1998).

Cross-Sectional Study: a snapshot of the presence of disease in a defined population at a given time (prevalence).

Systematic Review, and Meta-Analysis: a systematic review is methodical synthesis of empirical evidence fitting a pre-specified eligibility criteria, designed to answer a specific research question by using clearly defined systematic approach to limit bias and random error. A meta-analysis is a mathematical analysis of the combined results of two or more primary studies with similar designs, and often used in conjunction with the systematic review. For clear complete guidance on the use and scope of Systematic Reviews and Meta-Analysis, visit the National Institute for Heath Research Centre for Reviews and Dissemination based at York University and download their free comprehensive guide (**www.york.ac.uk/inst/crd/guidance.htm**) or access the Cochrane Collaboration handbook (**www.cochrane-handbook.org**).

Cohort Study: a longitudinal (prospective or retrospective) observational study to examine to possible relationship between exposure to a risk factor and the development of disease. Participants are grouped based on exposure to a particular risk factor, and followed up to find association with the development of disease, and the natural history of disease.

Case-Control Study: a longitudinal observational study examining the relationship between the development of disease and past exposure to a risk factor. Participants are grouped as those with or without a disease, and prior exposure to a certain risk factor is then investigated.

Ecological Studies: a population-based observational study used to examine the distribution of disease between populations in relation to various risk factors.

Randomised Control Trial: a prospective experimental study in which participants are allocated at random to receive one of several clinical interventions (placebo, standard treatment, novel treatment, no treatment). Participants may be blinded to reduce bias. In single-blinded studies the participants are unaware of the therapy they receive. In double-blinded studies both the participants and the researcher are unaware of the treatment received.

Animal (in vivo) and In Vitro Experimental Studies: biomedical laboratory-based basic, applied, experimental, or translational research. Such studies generate new knowledge, develop new treatments, or test the efficacy, toxicity and pharmacokinetics of novel therapies in the preclinical setting.

Basic statistics

Try to become comfortable with basic statistics. A refresher course or friendly statistician will get you started. The cornerstones of health research are knowledge of variable types and summary measures (see Table 16.4), and of calculating the accuracy of diagnostic tests (see Table 16.5). The Centre for Evidence Based Medicine (CEBM. net) is again a good place to become familiar with important concepts such as using the 2 × 2 table, Risk, Odds, Numbers Needed to Treat (NNT), and P-values.

Microsoft Excel is most familiar spreadsheet format for collating your data, but open office (openoffice.org) is free and just as good. Many would recommend putting your data straight into PASW (Predictive Analytics SoftWare). Formerly

SPSS, PASW will process most statistical requests from simple medians and means up to regression analysis, statistical modelling, and beyond. A training course or guidebook on PASW is a worthwhile investment. Many open-source free statistical packages do exist of variable quality and usability (**www.statpages.org/javasta2. html#Freebies**).

Table 16.4 Variable types, summary measures and measures of spread

Type	Sub-Type	Appropriate Summary Measure	Appropriate Measure of Spread
Categorical	*Nominal* Arbitrary categories, e.g. gender	Mode	
	Ordinal Ordered categories, e.g. likert scale	Mode Median	Range Inter-Quartile Range
Metric	*Discrete* Counted units (integers) on a numerical scale, e.g. number of patients	Mode Median Mean	Range Inter-Quartile Range Standard Deviation
	Continuous continuous values on a numerical scale, e.g. duration of symptoms	Mode Median Mean	Range, Inter-Quartile Range Standard Deviation

Table 16.5 Assessing the accuracy of diagnostic tests

Term	Definition
True Positive (TP)	A test result is positive when the disease is present
False Positive (FP)	A test result is positive when the disease is not present
True Negative (TN)	A test result is negative when the disease is absent
False Negative (FN)	A test result is negative when the disease is present
Sensitivity: TP/(TP+FN)	The probability that the test will be positive when a person has the disease. A sensitivity of 100% means all positive patients were identified as positive
Specificity: TN/(TN+FP)	The probability that the test will be negative in a person without the disease. A specificity of 100% means all negative patients were identified as negative
Positive Predictive Value (PPV): TP/(TP+FP)	Proportion of people with a positive test with the disease
Negative Predictive Value (NPV): TN/(TN+FN)	Proportion of people with a negative test without the disease

Ethics, consent, and safety

Don't expect that you will be covered by your supervisors' ethics approval. Application processes for ethical approval can be time consuming and lengthy, take care to find out what you can do, and for what you will need additional ethical approval for from day one. Get in touch with your local Research and Development (R&D) department and ask them for local guidance regarding the conduct and practice of research, audit, and service evaluation. Below are some of the key documents that give important orientation on consent, ethics, safety and legislation detailed in the UKFPO Compendium of Academic Competencies.

Comprehensive guidance on gaining informed consent, the design of consent forms and information leaflets, and on gaining consent in adults unable to consent for themselves can be found on the UK National Research Ethics Service website (**www.nres.npsa.nhs.uk/applications/guidance**). There is also guidance on a wide range of topics such as phase 1 trials, clinical trials, the use of human tissue and of personal data.

All confidential patient identifiable data must be kept behind a trust or university firewall, saved in an encrypted password protected file (see Chapters 10 and 11). Any data taken offsite should be further anonymised. Be careful to back-up your files, keeping versions at key steps along the way to revert back to if data is lost, or corrupted.

For ethics and safety, the Medical Research Councils (MRC) guide to Good Research Practice is a readable run through of best practice. Whilst primarily written for laboratory scientists, it remains relevant to all (**www.mrc.ac.uk/Utilities/Documentrecord/index.htm?d=MRC002415**).

The legal framework for ethical study design and for the conduct and recording of research involving humans for investigational medicinal products is extensive found in the Good Clinical Practice Guidelines produced by the International Conference on Harmonisation of Technical Requirements for Registration of Pharmaceuticals for Human Use (ICH) (**www.ich.org**).

UK legislation surrounding the Medicines for Human Use (Clinical Trials) Regulations 2004 can be found at **www.legislation.gov.uk/uksi/2004/1031/contents/made** with the statutory instrument transposing this into UK Law on 29 August 2006 found at **www.legislation.gov.uk/uksi/2006/1928/contents/made**.

Funding

The best website to get a feel for the sort of funding out there is **www.rdinfo.org.uk**. RDInfo lists funders by organisation, funding streams and research areas and provides detailed advice and guidance on how to work through your funding application.

Dissemination

Visit **www.icmje.org** to access the uniform requirements for manuscripts submitted to biomedical journals. Read carefully about peer review, authorship and contributions, conflicts of interests, and acknowledgements. Choose your submission journal carefully reading their specific advice for authors. Most journals will have an online submission system through which the journal will communicate with you. If asked to review and resubmit your manuscript, respond to the reviewers comments keeping a step-by-step document detailing how you addressed each of their points, and submit this with your revised manuscript. Be patient and prepared to resubmit elsewhere, as persistence pays off.

Referencing

Referencing is easy with a reference manager, and choosing your desired output style with a simple click. EndNote, whilst the old faithful, is expensive. A subsidised limited warranty version will most likely be available through your university or NHS trust. The trick is to gather and index your journal articles as you go to save time when writing up. Some of the free open-source programs such as Zotero (Zotero. org), a plug-in for the open-source Firefox browser (mozilla.com), are feature laden, allowing for example indexing of articles direct from Pubmed into your library. A hunt online is worthwhile before starting your literature search.

Posters and presentations at conferences need not be daunting. Give yourself plenty of time to write and practise them pre-empting any questions you could be asked. Remember, you are the expert on your piece of research, so be confident. The internet is a great place to start looking at which conferences to attend, and your supervisor will know the best ones to prepare for. There are many scholarships available for junior researchers, so look out for these.

Chapter summary

This chapter has:

- summarised the knowledge and skills needed to get started with your research;

- offered case studies and activities to help you apply your understanding of research activities;

- provided links, resources, and strategies to help you meet the expectations set out in the UKFPO Foundation competencies and the Compendium of Academic Competencies.

GOING FURTHER

Bowers, D, House, A and Owens, D (2006) *Understanding Clinical Papers*, 2nd edition. Chichester: Wiley Publishing.

A practical guide to understanding clinical papers – aims to explain the important elements found in clinical research papers and how to interpret them.

Gordis, L (2009) *Epidemiology*, 4th edition. Philadelphia: Saunders Elsevier Publishing.
This book is an essential textbook for people studying epidemiology; it covers the key epidemiological concepts and methods.

Greenhalgh, T (2010) *How to Read a Paper: The Basics of Evidence-Based Medicine*, 4th edition. Oxford: Wiley-Blackwell Publishing.
This book offers guidance to reading medical papers, from basic level to more those studying at a higher level.

part 6
Working Effectively as a Professional

chapter 17

Managing Your Time and Workload
Sue Morgan and Liam Young

Achieving foundation competences

This chapter will help you to begin to meet the following requirements of the *Foundation Programme Curriculum* (2010).

Outcome 1 Professionalism

Practise with professionalism including: integrity; continuous improvement; aspiration to excellence

1.3 Time management and continuity of care

Competences
F1

- Is punctual for start of shifts, meetings, handovers and other duties.
- Keeps a list of tasks.
- Prioritises and re-prioritises workload appropriately.
- Delegates or calls for help in a timely fashion when s/he is falling behind.
- Ensures satisfactory completion of tasks at the end of the shift/day with appropriate handover.
- Makes adequate arrangements to cover leave.

F2

- Demonstrates an ability to adjust decision-making in situations where staffing levels and support are reduced (e.g. out of hours).
- Is aware of work pressures on others and takes appropriate action to help reorganise workloads.

3.10 Ensures safe continuing care of patients on handover between shifts, on-call staff or with 'hospital at night' team by meticulous attention to detail and reflection on performance

Competences
F1

- Attends handovers punctually and accepts directions and allocation of tasks from seniors.

F2

- Supports colleagues in forward planning at handover.
- Can, and sometimes does, organise handover, briefing and task allocation.
- Anticipates potential problems for next shift and takes pre-emptive action.

Outcome 14 Working with colleagues

Demonstrates effective teamwork skills within the clinical team and in the larger medical context.

14.1 Communication with colleagues and teamwork for patient safety

- F1 – displays understanding of personal role within the team and is able to support a team leader; listens to views of other healthcare professionals; meticulously cross-checks instructions and actions with colleagues (e.g. medicines to be injected); describes ways of identifying and dealing with poor performance in self and in colleagues.
- F2 – shows leadership skills where appropriate and at the same time works effectively with others towards a common goal.

14.2 Interface with different specialties and with other professionals

- F1 – shows an understanding of the challenges of providing optimum care within a variety of clinical settings; arranges appropriate urgent investigations and chases results when necessary.
- F2 – consistently seeks effective communication with colleagues in other disciplines.

Chapter overview

Throughout your medical career you will experience the tensions of what you *ought*, and what you would *like*, to be doing. One common way of dealing with job pressures is by working longer and harder but this comes at a considerable cost to our personal lives. In addition, the longer we work the less efficient we become and with the European Working Time Directive (EWTD) (see Directgov at **www.direct.gov.uk**) this option is no longer an open-ended one. At some point we cannot go on coping by just working longer.

This chapter gives some practical guidance on what you can do to prepare for your FY1 job and how to be an effective junior doctor. Strategies are described to enable smarter working so you can leave at the end of your shift with your jobs done, your patients safe and your training needs met.

After reading this chapter you should be able to:

- prepare adequately for your FY1 post, so are able to work to the expected level for your stage of training;
- prioritise your workload;
- ensure continuity of care for your patients within hospital and after discharge;
- ensure you meet your training needs;
- apply strategies to enable you to work smarter;
- practice tips to organise yourself;
- identify how to work co-operatively and get people to help you.

> Efficiency is doing things right. Effectiveness is doing the right things.
>
> (Drucker, 1993)

However slick and knowledgeable you are, if you have done the wrong job, you have failed, so this chapter will deal with these two items in reverse order.

Doing the right things

The first step in managing your time and workload is to have a clear idea of what your job includes.

Your key roles as a junior doctor are:

- patient care;
- your education;
- working in a team.

There will also be commitments to your employer and one of the key ones will be working with the terms of the EWTD. If trusts do not meet their terms, they are financially penalised so there will be considerable pressure on you to do your job in a timely fashion. The NHS web document 'Welcome to the Medical Team' (NHS Careers, 2010) gives a brief overview with many useful internet resources. The BMA's guidance 'Are you starting a new post?' (BMA, 2008) also provides a useful checklist.

Working hours

Junior doctor's hours are limited by two pieces of legislation:

- The UK Working Times Regulations (WTR – the UK version of the EWTD)
- The New Deal Contract.

European Working Time Directive

The EWTD has applied to junior doctors since August 2009 and states that:

- maximum working hours are 48 hours per week averaged over 17 weeks;

- you can opt out but this must be voluntary and in writing.

Even if you opt out, you cannot opt out of certain requirements of rest periods (minimum rest periods between shifts and breaks during shifts). Details can be found on the BMA website (**www.bma.org.uk**).

Be prepared

ACTIVITY 17.1 BEFORE YOU START YOUR JOB

- Contact the hospital and check what the induction arrangements are.
- If shadowing your predecessor is not included, set aside at least two days to do this including a period on call. This will save you a lot of stress and time later.
- Read the NHS Rough Guide to the Foundation Programme (2010) **www.foundationprogramme.nhs.uk/pages/foundation-doctors/key-documents**.
- Ensure you are familiar with your e-portfolio.
- Check what you need to organise in your first week for your education.
- Set yourself an initial target (not too ambitious) for example 1 DOP (Directly Observed Procedure) and 1 mini-CEX (Mini Clinical Evaluation Exercise) by the end of the first month and put them in your diary.

Patient care: facilitating your patient's journey through the hospital jungle

Your main duty is to care for your patient's needs and that they are safely discharged. In order to do this there are several key elements:

Treatment Phase

- Problem identification

- Diagnosis

- Investigation

- Treatment.

Recovery phase (fit for discharge)

- Nutrition

- Exercise.

Ensuring successful discharge

- Continuity treatment
  - Patient education
  - Discharge letter
  - Therapy.
- Continuity care
  - GP
  - Out-patients.
- Enabling
  - Home visit
  - Adaptations
  - Support – carers.

In order to do this effectively you need to know:

- Your patients
  - Who the patients are (name, age, diagnosis, social circumstances)
  - How well do they have to function in order to cope at home
  - What support may they need.

- Your hospital
  - Who does what
  - What services are available on site
  - Where and how to refer for other investigations.

- Your community
  - GPs
  - Support services.

Case study 17.1: The wind and the sun (adapted from Aesop's fable of the sun and the wind)

Dr Wynd and Dr Suun were FY1 colleagues each responsible for half of a busy medical ward. They would both go on the consultant round. Dr

Wynd had been top of his year passing with flying colours and winning prizes. Dr Suun had just scraped a pass, however he was well prepared.

On the ward round, Dr Wynd presented his patients with long lists of differential diagnoses, citing the latest research findings on each condition but failed to have a list of blood results, the urine dips had not been done and precious time was wasted getting each scan up. He had no idea of the patient's social circumstances as he was not interested and thought it wasn't his job. The consultant became increasingly frustrated and irate. No plans could be made and the ward round stretched on.

By the time Dr Suun presented, the consultant was not in a good humour. However despite Dr Suun's limited knowledge, he had a list of the blood results, scan reports were printed out and filed and he had tested the urine himself. He spent time chatting to his patients so he knew about their individual circumstances. The patients slipped by, the consultant warming more and more to Dr Suun. The round finished on time and the consultant slipped off his white coat and invited Dr Suun to join him in clinic. Dr Wynd meanwhile was left to run around chasing urine dips and taking bloods.

Organising and being organised is the main responsibility of the F1. This may *sound* easy but being organised is a skill and requires knowledge. It reduces 'faf' (finding another form). Faf can also manifest in looking for a blood bottle that is never kept on that ward.

ACTIVITY 17.2 SCOUTING FOR DOCTORS – BE PREPARED

Make a list of:

- any paper forms that you will potentially need – for example request forms, paper e-portfolio forms;
- 'tools' that you could require on the ward round – for example, peak flow meter;
- 'tools' you could require whilst on call – for example, phlebotomy or cannulation equipment.

Now decide, depending on your working environment, how you can best collate and store these items for yourself. For example, you may have a trolley with only your patient notes, in which case your forms and tools could all be kept here. If not, then invest in a suitable bag in which to carry it all. You may feel like a nerd wandering about with a bag all the time, but you'll be a nerd who goes home at 5 p.m.

Your education

Your next duty after ensuring your patients are cared for is your education. This does not have to be a formal teaching session – make the most of informal occasions. See Chapter 2 for ideas about how to get the best from your education. If tasks are planned over the course of a job, getting signed off is achievable. Do not leave all to the last month – you may fail one – and then you have no plan B.

In the *first week* of your placement you need to have:

- the educational agreement signed;
- the summary of educational review completed;
- the development plan completed.

Getting trained is a core part of being an F1 doctor, and ultimately it's up to you; if you don't get the Directly Observed Procedures (DOPS), Mini Clinical Evaluation Exercises (Mini-CEXs) and Case Based Discussions (CBDs), you don't get signed off. These can often be the bottom of your list of priorities on a day-to-day basis or even a firm-by-firm basis. Some people think they will make them up in the less busy jobs but that isn't the way to think about it. Get into the habit – view everyone as an assessor and everything as an assessment opportunity.

ACTIVITY 17.3 GET INTO THE HABIT

- Write down the staff who see you carrying out the most activities; remember for DOPS and some mini-CEX, these do not have to be doctors.
- Identify times when you are most likely to present cases to registrars or consultants as these are ideal times to ask for a mini-CEX.
- Put a note on your phone or paper diary to remind yourself to ask for DOPS or mini-CEXs on those days, remember to ask *before* the case as the assessor needs to know what they are assessing.
- Book a time with the consultant either directly or via their secretary to do a CBD right at the beginning of the rotation.

Doing things right

Don't underestimate the power of being organised and the simple list.
Ensure you are mentally and physically fit to do your job.

Get it right first time

- Check you understand what is being asked of you:
  - for example, rephrase the question or instruction back as you understood it and check the person agrees;

- get a timeframe for when it needs to be done by;
- if you don't understand why you are doing it, then ask – it's an educational opportunity.

- Try to avoid carrying out difficult tasks when you are tired by doing them first.

- Do any emotionally laden tasks first or set a time for these so you can focus on the rest of your workload.

- If something (e.g an e-mail, a request or a job) does not make sense to you in the light of what you already know, double check.

Where does your work come from and when?

If you understand where your work comes from and when this will happen, this allows you to plan your work much more effectively (Pedlar, 2001). Large batches of work commonly result from consultant rounds; if this is left until after the round, then you may still be on the ward until 8 p.m.

Pressure times

Although pressure times may occur unpredictably, many occur at set times, such as after ward rounds, at the end of shifts and on call.

Coping strategies

- Buddy up with a colleague – whilst one of you is presenting the other carries out tasks.

- Carry referral forms (see Activity 17.2) and complete them on the round.

- Predict – do as much as is sensible in advance of the round – for example, partially filled in blood request and X-ray forms.

- Have a suggested plan that the consultant can agree or amend.

- When covering, check the wards in quiet times. This has more than one payback:
  - networking with nursing staff;
  - gaining a reputation as a reliable worker;
  - building a relationship of trust buys you time, as the staff know you will come and they will chase less;
  - earn goodwill by lending a hand to others.

- Try and avoid chasing results (see below).

ACTIVITY 17.4 PRESSURE POINTS

- List the pressure times over the last week.
- How many were predictable and likely to recur?
- If yes to both, what can you do to avoid or relieve the pressure for next week?

Chasing referrals, investigations and results

Try to keep this activity to a minimum as it:

- wastes your time;

- irritates those being chased.

The main way to avoid chasing is to hone your technique in asking for the referral or investigation. Know the system so that you request in the right manner either electronically, via a proforma, a letter or book. Make urgent referrals in person (see Activity 17.5) or if a patient can be seen as an out-patient, ensure there is a copy of your letter in the front of the case notes. Do not irritate senior colleagues by neglecting this courtesy. The referral letter can be short:

- thank them for seeing the patient;

- ensure the reason for the review is clearly stated;

- highlight any particular concern;

- attach a copy of the discharge summary.

Referrals to senior colleagues

Although most referrals and requests are done electronically, urgent referrals should be done in person. Making a referral face to face can often feel daunting, so make sure you are fully prepared and work collegially with the person you are referring to, keeping the best interests of your patient at the forefront of what you are asking for.

ACTIVITY 17.5 REFERRALS AND REQUESTS

Make a list of the face-to-face referrals or requests you will commonly be making. List the generic information:

- name, DOB, ward;
- reason for admission;
- relevant past medical history.

Now for the various specialities make a list of what they specifically will ask. If you don't know, it is well worth asking the specialist registrar. For example, renal referral: baseline creatinine and urea, calcium, phosphate, urine dip, etc.

Note the question that needs answering and why it is urgent; for instance, what will change as a result. Ask your registrar or consultant if you don't know (often this can stump them too), and thereby save yourself the long walk back from the radiology department with a flea in your ear.

Situations that should be kept to the minimum

Being chased

- *Bleep* – make every effort to answer your bleep promptly and politely, saying who you are and your role if you don't know who is ringing you.

- *Request for task* – if you can't do it immediately, make it clear when you will do it so you do not have to answer the same call in an hour's time.

- *Relatives* – arrange to see them. If you can't answer their questions satisfactorily, either find out the answers or arrange for someone more senior to talk to them. Avoid multiple unsatisfactory interchanges.

Setting yourself up to fail

Know your expertise level. You may be able to have a go at a procedure, but unless you are competent, you risk damaging both patient and yourself. Sorting out the problem afterwards will take much longer and be more stressful. If you have not done the procedure for a while, you may need to be supervised again.

Complaints/errors

This may sound like a statement of the obvious – who in their right minds would wish to incur either? Thus having strategies in place to avoid errors are important and are not a waste of time. In addition, sometimes double checking what you have done before leaving a shift can defer anxiety. Complaints and errors consume vast amounts of time and emotional energy, frequently leaving us less resourceful.

- Pass dissatisfied patients/relatives upwards.

- Very occasionally you may have a complete empathy failure with a patient: if possible try to arrange for someone else to manage their care, otherwise you will inevitably try to avoid them, which will not enhance their care.

Losing your cool

If you are in an emotional turmoil, it is not easy to think and act logically and efficiently. Not only do you work slower but you make mistakes, which then take time to undo. Even worse, if you lose your temper, you may destroy carefully constructed relationships. There will always be people or things in your day which will cause you irritation. The art is minimising their impact. If you are in control, issues become less stressful. Try either taking time out or talking with a colleague, you may find they have the same problem or even have a solution. See Chapters 3 and 18 for ideas and strategies for reducing and dealing with stress.

Case study 17.2: The ant and the grasshopper (adapted from Aesop's fable of the ant and the grasshopper)

Dr Y, a cheerful if somewhat slightly vacant looking FY1, spent the entirety of his first two months wandering the corridors, saying hello to people he met in the far reaches of the hospital. His colleagues used to laugh and point at him, 'There goes Dr Livingston, discovering lost tribes of doctors, all his salary spent on shoe leather', or 'Poor guy, apparently he has fingers the size of milk bottles and can't use a phone'. However, as the winter drew in and the other FY1s became busier and busier and winter wards opened to accommodate all the admissions, Dr Y was not frantically scurrying about seeing patients all over the hospital. He didn't have to stand in a queue of human marshmallows waiting to be toasted by a consultant radiologist on why their scan was not urgent whatever their consultant thought.

Why? Well in the first two months when he had more time, he had spoken to the secretaries that booked the scans, stopped for coffee, taken biscuits or shared out chocolates that patients had given him. He found out from the bed managers what information helped them to decide where the patients went. These people knew him by name and face and liked the fact that he had given them his time and interest. This meant that when the busy times came, he could get on the phone and say 'Hi, it's me' and they knew who he was and nine times out of ten said they 'would do it *for him*'. His patients went to the wards he wanted them to go to; his scans got squeezed into slots. He didn't need to keep walking the corridors as much, his colleagues didn't laugh at him any more, they didn't point either, though they did wave goodbye as he left at 5 p.m.

ACTIVITY 17.6 MANAGING YOUR EMOTIONAL RESPONSE

List two or three episodes in your work or leisure that have irritated or upset you over the last week.

For each, answer the following questions:

- What happened?
- What was it that caused the aggravation?
- Was my emotional response in proportion to the problem?
- Will it or a similar issue be likely to occur again?
- What was my part in contributing to the problem?
- Could this be prevented in the future by taking action now? If so what steps should I take?

Ways you may sabotage yourself by time wasting

Emotional sabotage

This may include agonising over, rather than making decisions about problem patients, mistakes or your future career choices. You might also let anger interfere with decisions or work when fatigued, which may result in disengagement with the job, with patients and with colleagues.

Procrastination using diversional activities

This might involve doing easier tasks and then running out of time or energy to do important tasks or doing tasks that are completely unrelated to getting the job done.

Do dirty

Here you might complete the task fast and badly, knowing it has been done inadequately.

Pass the buck

This can include leaving a job for the next shift to do although it was your responsibility to sort this out.

Forget

You might conveniently forget to carry out a task so you not have to deal with the emotions involved in acknowledging one has not done this well (can stem from feelings of personal inadequacy) and the need to ask for help from another.

Fail to ask for help

Here you have no clear idea of the nature of the problem with a patient and no clear plan. Instead of asking for help, unnecessary tests are arranged and the patient deteriorates before the necessary advice is sought.

Time management tips

One of the ways to manage your time and prioritise is to use a time management matrix, which divides tasks into urgent or important. The Businessballs™ website provides many self-management activities and suggests that deciding whether activities are urgent, important, both or neither, is crucial for good time management. Table 17.1 gives examples of tasks which fit into each of the quadrants in the time management matrix.

Most inexperienced people, and people who are not good at time management, nor in managing their environment, tend to spend most of their time in boxes 1 and 3.

Table 17.1 Time management matrix

	Urgent	*Not urgent*
Important	1 DO NOW	2 PLAN TO DO
	• emergencies, complaints and crisis issues • demands from superiors or patients • planned tasks or work now due • meetings and appointments • reports and other submissions • staff/patient issues or needs • problem resolution, fire-fighting, fixes Subject to confirming the importance and the urgency of these tasks, do these tasks now. Prioritise according to their relative urgency.	• planning, preparation, scheduling • educational tasks and learning • research, investigation, designing, testing • networking relationship building • thinking, creating, modelling, designing • systems and process development • anticipation and prevention • developing change, direction, strategy Critical to success: planning, strategic thinking, deciding direction and aims, etc. Plan time-slots and personal space for these tasks.

Not important	3 REJECT AND EXPLAIN	4 RESIST AND CEASE
	• trivial requests from others • apparent emergencies • ad-hoc interruptions and distractions • misunderstandings appearing as complaints • pointless routines or activities • accumulated unresolved trivia • boss's whims or tantrums Scrutinise and probe demands. Help originators to re-assess. Wherever possible reject and avoid these tasks sensitively and immediately.	• 'comfort' activities, computer games, net surfing, excessive cigarette breaks • chat, gossip, social communications • daydreaming, doodling, over-long breaks • reading nonsense or irrelevant material • unnecessary tidying or adjusting of equipment etc. • embellishment and over-production Habitual 'comforters' not true tasks. Non-productive, de-motivational. Minimise or cease altogether. Plan to avoid them.

Note: Adapted from the Urgent and Important Time Management Matrix at **www.businessballs.com/timemanagement.htm** (accessed 1 January 2011).

Poor time managers tend to prioritise tasks (and thereby their time), according to who shouted last and loudest (loudness often correlates to seniority, which discourages most people from questioning and probing the real importance and urgency of tasks received from those above them). Spare time is typically spent in box 4, which comprises only aimless and non-productive activities. Most people spend the least time of all in box 2, which is the most critical area for success, development and proactive self-determination. Source is **www.businessballs.com/timemanagement.htm** (accessed 1 January 2011).

Box 17.1 Time management tips

- When you're faced with a pile of things to do, go through them quickly and make a list of what needs doing and when. After this, handle each piece of paper only once. Do not under any circumstances pick up a job, do a bit of it, then put it back on the pile. Do not start lots of jobs at the same time.
- Be absolutely firm in dealing with time allocated for meetings, paperwork, telephone, and visitors.
- Review your work environment, layout, IT equipment, etc., and set it up for efficiency. Tidy up your work-space and keep all paperwork filed away unless you're

working on it. Keep a clean desk and well-organised systems, but don't be obsessive, or spend all week adjusting the settings of your screen-saver.

- Delegate as much as possible to others whilst still ensuring you do what you are required to.
- If you can't stop interruptions, go elsewhere when you need time alone. Fight for your right to work uninterrupted when you need to.
- Sharpen up your decision-making. If you can't decide, decide how to (e.g. consult, get more information, delegate, etc.), but don't just let it sit there.
- Learn to say 'No', politely, and constructively. Don't make a rod for your own back. Be careful about accepting sideways delegation by your peers to you. If you find it difficult to say 'No', you'll find it easier by using patient care reasons to justify your position.
- Always probe deadlines to establish the true situation – people asking you to do things will often say 'now' when 'later today' would be perfectly acceptable.
- Never try to eat an elephant all in one go, (i.e. break very big tasks down into digestible chunks). Use project management techniques for large jobs.

Adapted from **www.businessballs.com/timemanagement.htm**.

Prioritising in the clinical environment

The time management matrix and other tips described above will help you manage your time in general but when faced with multiple tasks in the clinical environment you must prioritise them more quickly and this rests on your developing clinical judgement as well as other skills such as communication and leadership. However, you can only prioritise as important or urgent (or neither) if you have sufficient information.

- Ensure the referrer gives you the necessary information and observations.

- If you decide that more than one patient needs assessing immediately, call for help sooner rather than later.

- If a patient can wait to be seen after a more acute case, ensure the referring staff have a clear idea of what they should be doing until you arrive in terms of observations and treatment. This deals with the referrer's anxiety that they are behaving appropriately.

Delegating

The most effective way of saving time is by delegating work to others and getting to know the people who can save you time should not be underestimated (see Case

Study 17.2). As an F1 doctor, this will often be by negotiation rather than straight delegation but buddying up with colleagues can be a useful strategy. However, you need to bear in mind that although an issue (such as asking for an observation) may be top of your priority list, others may have competing demands on their time.

When do you need it done by?

- Now – do it yourself.

- Within x minutes – check nursing staff will be able to do this – if you need to chase them to do it, it will be quicker for you to do than delegate.

Check your requests have been carried out

Fluids

If it is very important that your patient is adequately rehydrated then:

- write up adequate amount, to be given fast enough;

- see that the line is set up and fluids running before you leave the ward – this may mean you do it yourself;

- tell the named nurse when the bag should be through so it can be monitored, not discovered eight hours later when the bag finally empties;

- go back and check fluids in the patient. If they have run slow, you may need to revise the schedule you have written.

Drugs

- Write up.
- Check they are on the ward.
- Observe the first dose given.

This may sound obsessive but it is quicker to get things right the first time. When treatment is critical, it is best to be obsessive. The consequences, if treatment is not done in a timely fashion, may be serious.

- Your patient may be harmed.

- A sicker patient will take more of your (and everyone else's) time.

- An emotional cost will be paid by your feelings of guilt, your boss's reduced confidence in you and a loss of trust from patient and relatives.

- A financial cost to the NHS and possibly to the patient will be incurred.

The responsibility for the treatment being carried out in a timely fashion is yours.

Continuity of care

The EWTD has forced shift working onto the medical profession. This has the enormous benefit of doctors not being worked beyond their limits but can come at considerable cost if adequate systems are not in place. In particular, adequate training opportunities and continuity of care have to be addressed.

Your patients are your responsibility. In order to finish your shift, you need to ensure to the best of your ability that they will be safe until you return. This requires a clear understanding of the investigation and treatment plan for each patient.

What tasks do you need to do or handover before leaving the hospital?

- Chasing results – ensure your blood tests are done early to keep this to a minimum, for example:

  - Potassium level in a hyperkalaemic patient, this needs to be checked as you may alter the treatment in response to this.

  - Digoxin level – ensure next day's digoxin is not given on drug chart until you have had time to review result.

- Completing tasks on a patient you have handed over to another team – be clear on your hospital policy where your responsibility ends. Ensure that there is no gap in the continuity of the patient's care and that the next team has accepted the care of that patient, document in the notes and ensure the ward staff have been informed.

- Routine tasks on your patients should be completed wherever possible:

  - Writing up warfarin.

  - Writing up fluids – note that you may need to get your patient reviewed.

Handover meetings

Ensure you have a clear plan for these meetings.

- Written/electronic list of patients you need to have reviewed.

- What the next shift needs to review?

- How often they need reviewing?

- What action do they need to take if the patient deteriorates?

- Who needs to review this patient? Can a F1/2 doctor review or do they need more senior review?

- Will that person be at the handover meeting?

- Yes – as bulleted above.

- No – track them down beforehand – if they are not available because they are in theatres then you can carry out a Plan B – for example, refer to Surgical FY1 with clear steer to get his senior to review, providing written information as above. If the review is urgent, get the SHO out of theatres.

For more on handover and communication with colleagues, patients and relatives, see Chapters 7, 8 and 13.

Discharge letters

Your patients' care needs to continue in the community. Consider what their GP needs to know about their hospital admission in order to do this. Highlighting the key pieces of information when writing the notes can make this task easier.

Discharge letters act as an invoice for the PCT. If various treatments, co-morbidities and complexities of the case are not included, the extra costs incurred are not paid. This can mean significant amounts of money being lost by your trust. Not many employers would tolerate a worker who sent out a bill and only charged for half the work that was done.

They also play a key role in information stored on databases. Thus inaccurate recording of information may lead to inaccurate research conclusions and ultimately healthcare planning.

Chapter summary

This chapter has covered the following topics which will enable you to:

- Do the right things – know what your job consists of and the demarcation of duties.

- Do things right – simple methods to ensure effective working and that you complete in a timely fashion to meet EWTD.

- Know who can make your life easier.

- Identify and avoid less effective behaviours.

- Use time management techniques to simplify and order your work and home life.

- Make your training a top priority by building it into part of your working life. Start immediately and have a clear plan with timelines and diary reminders.

- Ensure continuity of care for your patients.

GOING FURTHER

Forsyth, P *Successful Time Management*, revised 2nd edition. The Sunday Times Audiobook.

Allen, D (2008) *Getting Things Done*. London: Piatkus. The advantage over the audiobook is that you can skip the less relevant passages. The joy of this book is the quotes that are used alongside the text, for example: 'I am rather like a mosquito in a nudist camp; I know what I want to do but I don't know where to begin' (Stephen Bayne).

chapter 18

Self-management

Charlie Cooper

Achieving foundation competences

This chapter will help you to begin to meet the following requirements of the *Foundation Programme Curriculum* (2010).

Outcome 1 Professionalism

Practise with professionalism including: integrity; compassion; altruism; continuous improvement; aspiration to excellence; respect of cultural and ethnic diversity; regard to the principles of equity; ethical behaviour; probity (refer to GMC *Fitness to Practise* declaration in F1 and *Standards for Training for the Foundation Programme* in *The New Doctor*).

1.1 Behaviour in the workplace

Competences

- Always recognises own level of competence and asks for help from appropriate sources.
- Demonstrates the ability and habit of reflection on experience, as well as learning from practice, then instituting appropriate changes in this practice.
- Acts with empathy, honesty and sensitivity in a non-confrontational manner.
- Respects and supports the privacy and dignity of patients.
- Is courteous, polite and professional when communicating with both patients and colleagues.
- Has a non-judgemental approach.
- Is aware of patient expectations around personal presentation of doctors such as dress and social behaviour.
- Encourages an atmosphere of open communication and appropriately directed communication within teams.
- Recognises the potentially vulnerable patient, for example, children, older people, those in need of extra support.
- Only shares clinical information, whether spoken or written, with appropriate individuals or groups.
- Seeks out role models and tries to learn from the behaviours of the best clinical practitioners and leaders.

1.2 Health and handling stress and fatigue

Competences

- Where relevant, takes responsibility for ensuring that personal or others' health, does not compromise that of colleagues or patients.

Knowledge

- The risks to patients if one's own performance is compromised by health problems.
- The effects of stress and/or fatigue on performance.
- The circumstances when self-referral to occupational health services are appropriate.
- The availability of support facilities.

Outcome 14 Working with colleagues

- Demonstrates effective teamwork skills within the clinical team and in the larger medical context.

14.1 Communication with colleagues and teamwork for patient safety

- F1 – displays understanding of personal role within the team and is able to support a team leader; listens to views of other healthcare professionals; takes leadership role and delegates appropriately in the context of own competence; describes ways of identifying and dealing with poor performance in self and in colleagues.

The chapter will also introduce you to some of the Leadership and Management outcomes set out in the *Compendium of Academic Competencies* published by the UK Foundation Programme Office and the *Medical Leadership Competency Framework* (Academy of Medical Royal Colleges and the NHS Institute for Innovation and Improvement, 2010). See Chapter 14 for more on leadership and management

Chapter overview

Samuel Smiles published *Self-Help with Illustrations of Character and Conduct* in 1859. In his second edition, Smiles included the word 'perseverance' at the end of the title (Smiles, 1866). In this chapter, entitled 'Self-management', you will discover that perseverance, coupled with looking after yourself, is a key attribute of the successful and content doctor. It is not an accident that the General Medical Council (GMC) has chosen to prioritise its first statement concerning Conduct, that

F1 doctors 'must demonstrate that they are able to take appropriate action if their own health, performance or conduct, . . . puts patients, colleagues or the public at risk' (General Medical Council, 2009c, pp5–7).

The previous chapters in this book have described the key generic aspects of postgraduate education, training and professional development required of a foundation trainee. In this concluding chapter, these have been brought together within the theme of managing yourself. This is dealt with under several headings, the first is 'Self-insight' which was discussed in depth in Chapter 3.

After reading this chapter you will be able to:

- recognise that you must take responsibility for your well being and your behaviour;
- recognise the signs of positive and negative stress in yourself and others;
- know when to ask for help and where it can be found;
- identify the daily requirement for honesty (probity) in self-reflection and therefore in your interaction with others;
- recognise the importance of taking time to talk and think things through.

Self-insight

This is the key component to managing yourself. It might well be that because others know we need support, we are already receiving gentle advice from those around us without realising it. Paying attention to these cues from others can be an invaluable early clue that we are not managing ourselves as well as we could and that our self-insight is not as reliable as we had thought or hoped. Bearing this in mind, try Activity 18.1.

ACTIVITY 18.1 PERFORMANCE AND CONDUCT

Download and read the 'For the record' article entitled 'Doctor's performance and conduct fall short of standards expected' on p15 of the November/December 2009 edition of the GMC publication, GMC today – **www.gmc-uk.org/publications/5047.asp**.

What might have been the underlying causes of this doctor's poor attendance records at work and training meetings?

Get organised

Becoming disorganised may explain a feeling of being perpetually one step behind where you want to be. The relevant time management strategy to maximise personal organisation is the prioritisation of tasks. Chapter 17 provides a range of strategies for time management and prioritising. Working collaboratively with others is as much about the little things such as asking for help as it is about mustering senior assistance in a crisis. Chapters 7, 8 and 13 cover many aspects of team working, collaboration and communication skills.

ACTIVITY 18.2 REFLECTING ON FEEDBACK

Have you ever 'played down' a worry or concern about yourself without meaningful reflection? If so, spend ten minutes reflecting on the reasons that led you to under-value the importance of the feedback – write them down.

Every aspect of daily life will benefit from a discrete improvement in organisational management, so do not neglect your home environment, your friends and of course your family when you review how you run your day-to-day activities. Use the time management matrix described in Chapter 17 to identify areas where you might improve your time management. Improvements in organisational management reliably improve our working environment and therefore our well-being, often without requiring new and unachievable skills. Activity 18.2 is important; honestly completing this seemingly innocuous activity may prove more difficult than you initially anticipate. Understanding and then overcoming prevarication in our working environment is closely related to our approach to time management.

Take personal responsibility for yourself

Managing prevarication is part of a wider responsibility, namely to ensure that we are well motivated, both at home and at work. Prevaricators frequently rely on external factors, such as deadlines to motivate themselves and of course external factors can be an effective basis for motivation. But of greater importance is to look within oneself for the resources we use as a doctor and self-insight is a necessary prerequisite.

Maintaining your self-motivation, your focus, requires an understanding of what it is that makes you choose to do something. Assertiveness is not just about one's approach to others, it is also about clarity and honesty during private self-reflection. Effective self-motivation will improve your confidence, your planning and the implementation of your decisions. It will also help those around you; in other words, it is an important contribution to your team (Trivedi et al., 2008). Activity 18.3 is an opportunity to explore these ideas.

ACTIVITY 18.3 WORKING EFFICIENTLY

Think of a colleague whose efficiency at work you admire and ask yourself if you know the secret of their efficiency; perhaps you know, perhaps you don't – you could always ask!

Now think of a colleague you work with and imagine they have asked you for advice on efficient ways of working. Now imagine what tips you would give them.

Finally, ask yourself whether you always follow your own advice. What are the real reasons you don't follow your own advice?

Manage your physical well-being

Most of us enjoy good health most of the time and soon recover when we are ill. Remember, it is OK to admit to being ill, it happens to us all! Maintaining good physical and mental health is predicated upon a good diet, effective rest and keeping physically fit. Working hard and getting tired are a normal part of a healthy lifestyle.

We all interact with friends and family and many of us have partners. Take time to discuss the requirements you each have for a happy life and recognise that, just as your partner may not have insight into your own needs, alarmingly, the opposite may instead be true. We know things about others that they do not seem to know themselves, the reverse is also generally true – back to self-insight then. The Johari Window exercise in Chapter 3 can help you provide insight into how you and others see yourself.

Start looking after your health by registering with a GP. You must not self prescribe: this is a GMC requirement. It is also unwise to ask colleagues to prescribe short-term treatment for you. It is straightforward to visit your GP or arrange an urgent telephone appointment. Really, it is.

Ill health

Ill health may or may not lead to a doctor getting into difficulty, but it is a risk factor. Seeking medical advice does require that an individual is aware they are ill; so that's back to self-insight again. Seeking feedback from friends or colleagues is not easy, for reasons of both confidentiality and, frankly, embarrassment. Review Case study 18.1 as an example of a serious illness that masqueraded as tiredness or exhaustion.

Occupational Health support will be available in your workplace – make use of it if necessary, it is confidential. Your occupational health physician is required to inform you and your employer if you are not fit for work and also to advise you and your employer of reasonable amendments or additions to the workplace that would allow you to work more effectively. Sometimes, more specialist occupational health support is required. This is accessed through your Deanery Office. A list of Deanery websites is available at **www.copmed.org.uk**.

If you know somebody who may be ill, or perhaps you are worried you may be, then it might be time to create a safe opportunity to ask or give feedback or advice. If you are unsure whether or not you are ill, pick a trusted person who knows you and then, if you can, sit down with them in a comfortable and safe place and say, 'I'm worried I may be ill' and then quietly listen. But, ultimately, if uncertain, you must consult your GP or occupational health physician.

Case study 18.1: Tired all the time?

Angela, an F2 had always been well. Then she noticed feeling 'deflated' about becoming less efficient. She wasn't making mistakes, although she was concerned she might be. She wisely saw her GP who asked a few questions about work, sleep patterns and diet and then agreed that an F2 job was much tougher than in her day. No formal advice was given.

Things got worse: poor sleep, weight gain and physical tiredness. Angela had stopped going out and hardly noticed she had ankle oedema. She visited the GP a couple more times, but didn't have the energy to confess the significance of her symptoms. Angela was literally at her wits end and felt as if she was 'going mad'.

Episodes of sick leave 'to cope' encouraged a medical friend to go with Angela to her GP. A blood test diagnosed hyperthyroidism.

Following treatment, Angela's life was transformed. Two things astounded Angela on her initial return to work: how pleased everybody was to see her and that nobody at work had noticed how ill she was. Her medical friends remain guilty that they didn't intervene earlier.

Your behaviour: probity

Good Medical Practice (General Medical Council, 2006) and *The New Doctor* (General Medical Council, 2009d) both set out with terse clarity the standards of personal behaviour that all GMC registered practitioners are required to maintain at all times, not just in the workplace. The reasons patients and their families accord doctors as a group the extraordinary privilege of responsibility for patients' health hinge on their doctor's behaviour, whatever their health outcome. The intertwining of doctors' maintenance of the highest standards of behaviour with the privileges bestowed on registered doctors in return enfolds medical regulation in the UK. Activity 18.4 is essential for foundation trainees.

> ## ACTIVITY 18.4 PROFESSIONAL STANDARDS
>
> Read the GMC publication Good Medical Practice (2009):
>
> **www.gmc-uk.org/guidance/good_medical_practice/duties_of_a_doctor.asp.**
>
> And read *The New Doctor* (2009):
>
> **www.gmc-uk.org/New_Doctor09_FINAL.pdf_27493417.pdf.**
>
> As you do so, reflect on the standards of behaviour mandated for the retention of your registration.

It is all too easy to give no more than a cursory thought to 'probity' as a new doctor; after all, you might feel it just means 'don't lie'. However, probity, as it refers to a GMC registered doctor, relates directly to the following wide range of personal behaviour, both in and outside the workplace:

- being honest: honest with yourself, your patients and others;
- integrity: doing the 'right' thing and sticking to it under pressure – includes financial integrity;
- being trustworthy: doing what you agreed to do;
- acting ethically: taking care to consider an individuals rights and circumstances; communicating openly; ensuring informed consent; declaring conflicts of interest;
- acting within the law: including communication to the correct authority when you become aware of an illegal act that could cause harm;
- acting so as to protect vulnerable individuals: including children;
- if you are concerned you may pose a risk to patients or staff, choosing not to rely solely on your own assessment of the risk;
- being alert to and acting upon the need to delegate, refer or ask for help.

Case study 18.2: Speaking up

Jane, an F2 in anaesthetics with a job interview coming up for an ST3 anaesthetics post, undertook a preoperative assessment for the consultant anaesthetist she was working with the next day. The operation was a short dental procedure requiring penicillin on induction. The patient's records covered two files; the first was missing. The patient denied any allergies; confirmed in the available file.

The patient arrived in the anaesthetic room with both files and denied allergies. As anaesthesia was being induced by the consultant, Jane noticed the missing file on the shelf, but for some reason chose to say and do nothing. The penicillin was given and the patient had an anaphylactic reaction.

Later, the first file revealed the penicillin allergy; the patient recovered. Jane remains unsure why she didn't speak up. But she is certain of one thing: whatever else was going on in the anaesthetic room, failing to speak up was a failure of probity.

The concept of Human Factors as a way for healthcare teams to anticipate and manage stressful situations is beyond the scope of this chapter (see also Chapter 6 for more on Human Factors). If your interest is piqued by Case study 18.2, refer to the Clinical Human Factors Group's UK-based website for useful resources. This can be found at **www.chfg.org/index.htm**.

Your behaviour: stress management

Stress, as far as this chapter is concerned, is the response we perceive in a stressful environment and is a combination of physical and psychological reactions to a stressful situation. Stress responses can be described in three stages, where stage 1 stress is a positive, motivating response that enables you to (for example) perform well in an examination or sporting event.

Stage 1 healthy responses in a stressful situation might be:

a heightened sense of awareness;

a mild anxiety reflecting insight into the need to work well with your team;

a feeling of relief that now you are confronting a stressful situation, you are able to keep things simple, follow routine and ask for assistance with assertion;

a dry mouth, mild tachycardia and an wry recognition that you are sweating with a sense that this is to be expected;

soon after the stressful moment has passed, a sense of satisfaction in sharing the experience (ethically) with openness, perhaps with colleagues you barely know;

later, perhaps that evening, falling to sleep easily with a sense of real achievement.

Less healthy, stage 2, responses to a stressful situation might be:

noticing you feel woolly-headed with difficulty ordering your thoughts;

feeling empty or distant from those around you;

feeling not so much anxious, as scared or perhaps being aware you may have 'blanked out' this emotion;

a realisation that now a stressful event has occurred, you feel an inner desire to try to leave and perhaps start rehearsing in your mind's eye ways of avoiding becoming too involved;

noticing that you feel mildly nauseated; perhaps also that your heart is pounding and, infuriatingly, you're sweating profusely;

sudden flashes of anger when something, perhaps a simple procedure goes awry. You may have no difficulty concealing them because of their brevity;

finding yourself being brusque or controlling in a group of peers;

shortly after a stressful event, a feeling of having let yourself down, despite doing well; perhaps a sense of discomfort in sharing your colleagues enthusiasm for chatting about the recent event;

later, perhaps that evening, having difficulty falling asleep or perhaps waking early, surprisingly alert, possibly with a mild sweat unsure why you woke. And then, shortly after, going back to sleep soundly until the alarm.

Many of us use 'comfort tricks' such as alcohol, food, smoking or procrastination to deal with stress and in the short term these can help provide a quick fix to a short-term problem. However, if stress continues, the comfort tricks can themselves become stressors (you will all have worked with patients who drink or smoke too much in response to stress) and a vicious cycle begins. It is important to self-monitor with regard to your own comfort tricks and use them to raise awareness of when your own stress levels are moving beyond those with which you can comfortably cope.

Stage 3 stress and burnout:

When stress becomes too much to bear and coping strategies stop working, people might move into stage 3 stress responses which can culminate (in the work situation) in 'burnout' or in a range of physical and psychological signs and symptoms which in extreme cases can contribute to heart disease, cancers, gastric disturbances and mental illness. Those who have either experienced or know of somebody who has had 'burnout', all agree that this is an alarming and distressing syndrome that is hard to overcome without considerable support at work and at home. The term 'burnout' refers to the consequences of long-term emotional exhaustion aligned with diminished interest (Maslach et al., 1996).

The consequences are best described in phases, which usually follow one after the other, leading to its most severe form (Kraft, 2006):

- a compulsion to prove oneself;
- working harder;
- neglecting one's own needs;
- displacement of conflicts – the person does not realise the root cause of the distress;
- revision of values – friends or hobbies are increasingly dismissed;
- denial of emerging problems – cynicism and aggression become apparent;
- withdrawal – reducing social contacts to a minimum, becoming walled off; alcohol or other substance abuse may occur;
- behavioural changes become obvious to others;
- inner emptiness;
- depression;
- burnout syndrome.

As Scott Boms (2009) suggests, it is important to remember the following to help tackle burnout:

- take time to chat and think things through – taking time is working;
- make time for yourself;
- get organised with a simple plan for a simple day – stick to your plan and always ask for help if you need it;
- set boundaries and expectations – these should be realistic, both for you and those around you. Write down reasonable and achievable goals that you and your friends would agree describe success;
- sleep – sleep more;
- if your situation needs to change, it can be changed safely;
- remain focused and beware undue distraction; remember that you're allowed to enjoy yourself!

The role of the educational supervisor and where to get help

All trainees have supervisors. The Educational Supervisor (ES) is responsible for induction, appraisal and feedback, including the written ES Report for each section of foundation training. Your ES should be approached to discuss matters of importance to you, so please make an appointment if you are worried, it will be in confidence (within the GMC guidelines for doctors on Confidentiality, 2009, paragraphs 35–36). You should make a written record of formal meetings with your ES, as should your ES. It is routine practice for the ES to set that out and, once agreed with you, both parties should sign. If, for some reason, you want to have a chat with somebody else, possibilities include your department College Tutor or Clinical Director or Trust Foundation Programme Lead or Director of Medical Education. Failing that, you would be expected to contact your Deanery's Foundation Programme Director or, if you wish, your Dean.

What to do if a doctor is in difficulty

This may or may not be you or somebody you know, either now or in the future. This chapter has assumed nothing about you because the points made are transferable and this is especially true for this last short section. There are two invaluable sources of information about this topic: the first is your Deanery (remember to look at the website) and the second is a National Association of Clinical Tutors (NACT) 2008 document entitled *Managing Trainees in Difficulty, Practical Advice for Educational and Clinical Supervisors*.

What exactly does the phrase 'doctor in difficulty' mean? The answer, without wishing to sound glib is: *there are as many answers as there are doctors in difficulty*. As a result, all the agencies involved in managing doctors in difficulty, whether that is the employer, the Deanery, the GMC or the National Clinical Assessment Service (for NCAS, visit **www.ncas.npsa.nhs.uk**), centre their advice on a process that is diagnostic. As a consequence, the first steps are gentle, make no assumptions and result in a first stage of equitable information gathering and support without judgement. The NACT guideline initially uses a diagnostic framework and then, if the concerns are substantiated, a management framework follows (NCAS, 2010). Two questions during the first phase are vital: 'Can they normally do it?' and 'Can they do it now?' Management then hinges on a consideration of how a difficulty can be allocated to one or more of four strands:

- clinical performance;
- personality and behavioural issues;
- health issues – physical and mental;
- environmental issues.

Remember that poor performance is not a 'diagnosis' but a symptom which requires exploration using the headings above. Remember also that patient safety is paramount and that documentation at every step is mandatory.

Chapter summary

Self-help is above all about self-insight and perseverance. This chapter has briefly covered a wide range of important topics that have arisen in other forms earlier in the book and all have self-insight and perseverance at their heart. In this chapter we have considered:

- the importance of self-insight;

- getting organised, time management and prioritising;

- taking personal responsibility;

- managing your physical and emotional well-being;

- probity;

- stress management and burnout

- the importance of asking for help when you (or others) need it and where to go for help

GOING FURTHER

Firth-Cozens, J (2003) Doctors, their wellbeing and their stress. *British Medical Journal*, 326: 670–71.

Lake, J (2009) Doctors in difficulty and revalidation: where next for the medical profession? *Medical Education*, 43(7): 611–12.

Maslach, C, Schaufeli, W and Leiter, M (2001) Job burnout. *Annual Review Psychology*, 52: 397–422.

McKimm, J (2009) Personal support and mentoring. In Cooper, N and Forrest, K (eds) *Essential Guide to Educational Supervision in Postgraduate Medical Education*, pp. 12–28. London: Wiley-Blackwell/BMJ Books.

McManus, I, Keeling, A and Paice, E (2004) Stress, burnout and doctors' attitudes to work are determined by personality and learning style. A twelve year longitudinal study of UK medical graduates. *BMC Medicine*, 2: 29.

BMA Doctors for Doctors Scheme: www.bma.org.uk/doctorsfordoctors (accessed 28 January 2011)

Windmills: www.windmillsonline.co.uk/ (accessed 28 January 2011)

Medical Careers: www.medicalcareers.nhs.uk/ (accessed 28 January 2011)

chapter 19

Becoming a Medical Professional: Change, Lifelong Learning and Professional Development

Judy McKimm and Kirsty Forrest

When you first start your working life as a doctor, it is an exciting though challenging time. After all, you have finally reached the goal that you have spent the last few years working hard towards. You have watched your non-medical friends leave university, and probably accumulated big debts, but you have achieved your aim of becoming a doctor. You may think that the biggest hurdle has been overcome by reaching the foundation stage of training but practising medicine is a continuous learning process and really the challenge is just beginning. Whichever speciality you are planning to enter, for up to ten years, there will always be 'just one more exam' and every day you will learn more: more about medicine, more about patients, and more about yourself.

Medical schools have always been very good at teaching students about the knowledge of diseases but not necessarily in preparing graduates for the practicalities of being a working professional practitioner. This is changing but the transition from student to doctor is still daunting. Many of the skills that aid this transition are explored in this book, based around the foundation curriculum, which includes both technical and non-technical skills.

In the introduction we set out the main aims of the book, which were to:

- assist the development of the knowledge, skills and competences required for good medical practice;

- address key areas within the 'generic', non-clinical elements and competences in the Foundation Programme to support professional practice;

- use case studies, activities and policy examples to illustrate key learning points;

- provide up-to-date information, reflect current policy developments and link to a range of useful information sources.

We hope that we have accomplished these aims and that you feel more informed and more 'practice ready' to work as a foundation doctor and beyond.

By now you are well aware that the knowledge and skills that make you into a good doctor are much more than knowing every disease and having a superb examination technique. It is vital that you display that somewhat elusive concept of 'being a professional' which the foundation curriculum and speciality curricula now set out in some detail in their competencies. Previously, the knowledge, skills and attributes that made doctors professional (the 'added extra') was learned by doctors over time. It was often implicit and many doctors learned the hard way, from mistakes which adversely affected patient care. We hope that for you the process of becoming professional started earlier, is much more explicit and that you are learning safely and not through error.

In this book, we have identified some core themes and issues which we discuss briefly in the next section in the light of changing medical practice.

Looking to the future

As in every walk of life, change is the only constant. Healthcare and medical education are no exceptions. It is important that you keep in touch with key bodies such as the General Medical Council (GMC), Medical Royal Colleges and deaneries so that you keep abreast with changes that could have serious implications for your education, training and future practice. For example, the GMC *Education Strategy 2011–2013: Shaping the Future of Medical Education and Training* (GMC, 2010d) sets out its key objectives for 2011–13 as follows:

- Setting and assuring standards, and valuing education and training.
- Promoting effective selection, transition and progression.
- Defining outcomes for education and training.
- Working with partners and promoting feedback and learning.

The GMC is now responsible for regulating all aspects of medical education and training from undergraduate through to postgraduate qualification and a much closer working relationship is being formed between the GMC, deaneries and local education providers (LEPs). As workforce deaneries move into a commissioning role, you will also see changes in the funding and structure of medical training and continuing professional development. Increasing expectations from all doctors includes an expansion of roles into teaching, supervision, research and management. All these roles are becoming more 'professionalised' and regulated. This places more pressure on clinicians who also have busy service commitments. Part of your development is learning how to juggle these roles and to identify what shape and balance of activities will suit you. There are many options available and seeking career advice both early on and when you feel at a crossroads is vitally important if you are to have a satisfying career.

In addition to regulatory and funding changes, wider developments in society will also impact hugely on access to and delivery of healthcare. The medical profession is still recovering from the impact of scandals such as Alder Hey, Bristol and Shipman which led to public inquiries that recommended that the medical profession is much more accountable to the wider public than it had been previously. For the individual practitioner, ensuring awareness of and keeping up to date with legal rules and professional guidance is essential in order to inform practice and cope with ethical dilemmas. It is important that you seek help if you feel you are struggling with any aspect of your practice, there are many support mechanisms available and you can be assured that you won't be alone or the first to have struggled.

New methods of training, assessment and revalidation have all been set in place to meet the need for more accountability and it will be important that the medical professional of the future is very aware of the need to maintain skills and knowledge and follow quality assurance processes. The GMC's website is continually being updated with new or revised version of key documents and interactive materials on selected topics (such as ethics). The NHS, deaneries, colleges and professional associations and other organisations all provide high-quality online training materials, journal articles are increasingly only available online and it is part of your professional responsibility to keep up to date in your field and be aware of how to access the right information in a timely fashion. As you work towards being an independent practitioner, structured training will lessen and so it is vital that you develop good lifelong learning skills and motivation. It will be important to keep good 'evidence' of training and development which will also increasingly rely on electronic records or portfolios. Appraisals and revalidation rely on evidence gathered from a range of sources, including peer and patient feedback, this means that you will also be required to support colleagues through providing feedback on their performance. The foundation stage assessments are all excellent preparation for such activities.

In this book, we aimed to set your professional practice within policy or strategy contexts with reference to supporting evidence that underlies practice wherever possible. The reason for this was twofold. First, we wanted to reflect contemporary health professional practice which needs to be grounded in evidence from research or evaluations of healthcare innovations and, second, we wanted to encourage you to always think about the wider context in which you are working. This wider context includes not only the organisation in which you work, but also the health system itself and then the wider societal and cultural context which influences healthcare delivery through funding, policy documents and the legal framework. Any clinical decision you make nearly always has a wider implication for you, the patient or the organisation and doctors have a key role to play in health management and leadership. Understanding the wider context will help you make more informed decisions, be more socially accountable and contribute more to your organisation and patient care. This wider role of the doctor is being emphasised internationally in terms of social accountability, and also by the GMC, for example in the new version of *Good Medical Practice* (General Medical Council, 2011).

As healthcare delivery is planned to move from hospital-based care to the community and the demography of society changes towards an increasingly ageing and multicultural society, the role of the doctor will need to change to meet health needs and expectations. The doctor's role is also changing with respect to other health professionals with extended scopes of practice becoming established in many professions as well as the emergence of new roles and professions. The need for doctors to work collaboratively as part of a multiprofessional team has been highlighted in policy documents and is reflected in interprofessional learning initiatives. Clinical decisions need to be supported by robust evidence, especially as funding is closely tied to evidence-based practice. Even if you are not involved in clinical research yourself, all doctors need to be able to interpret research findings and apply them to their own practice and will be involved in clinical audit. Involvement in audit and other governance activities also form part of the doctor's wider management responsibilities and responsibility for patient safety. You have seen the importance of ensuring safety and error reduction at the coalface, it is every clinician's responsibility to think about their role in system change to reduce errors and improve health outcomes. This again relies on understanding the evidence behind clinical decision-making and your responsibilities within health systems.

Technological advances in healthcare delivery will become more widespread. It is hard to predict how technology will impact on each speciality, but developments in pharmacology, nanotechnology, simulation, robotics, imaging, genetics and non-invasive therapies (to give just a few examples) have already changed the face of most branches of medicine. Health informatics developments, including patient records being held on electronic databases, will mean that health information will be more accessible and able to be shared more easily with other practitioners. This in turn may raise ethical issues which will need to be addressed.

Finally, at the heart of your professional practice is the relationship between you and patients. The nature of this relationship is also changing and is likely to change further as access to healthcare information via the internet and other media outlets widens and doctors are portrayed differently in the media and other public domains. What we are seeing is a renegotiation of what being a professional medical practitioner means. Patient empowerment movements and the way in which patients are seen as 'health partners' can at times feel challenging, even threatening, but the doctor–patient relationship is still vitally important in patient care. Good communication skills are intrinsically linked to professionalism. In recent years, communication skills have been the reason for the highest number of complaints about doctors in the UK. Patients assume doctors have the technical skills and knowledge to treat their disease or condition but want doctors who show they care for them and can communicate sensitively and appropriately. This has always been at the heart of being a good doctor, so although on the one hand massive changes are occurring specifically around the use of technology in medicine, the fundamentals of being a good 'professional' doctor remain as they always were: compassion, care and respect for patients.

To sum up, this book provides you with an overview of the various aspects of professional practice that doctors have to attend to in addition to clinical expertise. Although this all might seem daunting, your medical education to date should have prepared you well for integrating all these aspects into your day-to-day clinical practice and provided you with a sound foundation on which to enter speciality training. We hope that the case studies, examples and ideas in this book will support you on an exciting and fulfilling medical career which helps you to provide the best care for patients and carers that you can.

References

Academy of Medical Educators (2009) *Professional Standards*. London: Academy of Medical Educators. www.medicaleducators.org/index.asp (accessed 19 August 2010).

Academy of Medical Royal Colleges (2008) *A Code of Practice for the Diagnosis and Confirmation of Death*. www.aomrc.org.uk/aomrc/admin/reports/docs/DofD-fi nal. pdf.

Academy of Medical Royal Colleges (2009) *Common Competences Framework for Doctors*. London: Academy of Medical Royal Colleges. www.aomrc.org.uk/publications/reports-guidance.html (accessed 19 August 2010).

Academy of Medical Royal Colleges and the NHS Institute for Innovation and Improvement (2008a) *Engaging Doctors in Leadership: What Can We Learn from International Experience and Research Evidence?* www.institute.nhs.uk/medicalleadership (accessed 30 September 2010).

Academy of Medical Royal Colleges and the NHS Institute for Innovation and Improvement (2008b) *Engaging Doctors: Can Doctors Influence Organizational Performance?* www.institute.nhs.uk/medicalleadership (accessed 30 September 2010).

Academy of Medical Royal Colleges and the NHS Institute for Innovation and Improvement (2010) *Medical Leadership Competency Framework*. www.institute.nhs.uk/medicalleadership (accessed 29 August 2010).

Adair, J (1973) *Action-Centred Leadership*. New York: McGraw-Hill.

Baille WF, Buckman R, Lenzi R, Glober G, Beale EA and Kudelka AP (2000) SPIKES – A six-step protocol for delivering bad news: application to the patient with cancer. *The Oncologist*, 5 (4): 302–311.

Balarajan, R (1991) Ethnic differences in mortality from ischaemic heart disease and cerbrovascular disease in England and Wales. *British Medical Journal*, 302: 560–564.

Balarajan, R and Soni Raleigh, V (1993) *The Health of the Nation: Ethnicity and Health, a Guide for the NHS*. London: Department of Health.

Balarajan, R and Soni Raleigh, V (1995) *Ethnicity and Health in England*. London: HMSO.

Bass, B and Avolio, B (1994) *Improving Organisational Effectiveness through Transformational Leadership*. Thousand Oaks, CA: Sage.

Beauchamp, TL and Childress, JF (2001) *Principles of Biomedical Ethics* (5th edition). Oxford: Oxford University Press.

Bell, MDD (2007) The legal framework for end of life care: a United Kingdom perspective. *Intensive Care Med*, 33: 158–162.

Bell, MDD (2010a) GMC guidance on end of life care: important changes for clinicians take effect on 1 July. *BMJ*, 340: 1373–1374.

Bell, MDD (2010b) Emergency medicine and organ donation: a core responsibility at a time of need or threat to professional integrity. *Resuscitation*, 81 (9): 1061–1062.

Benning, A, Dixon-Woods, M, Ghaleb, M, Suokas, A, Dawson, J, Barber, N et al. (2011) Large scale organisational intervention to improve patient safety in four UK hospitals: mixed method evaluation. *British Medical Journal*, 342: d195.

Berwick, D and Leape, LL (1999) Reducing errors in medicine. *British Medical Journal*, 319: 136–137.

Bhabra, G, Mackeith, SPM and Pothier, DD (2007) An experimental comparison of handover methods. *Annals of The Royal College of Surgeons of England*, 89 (3): 298–300.

Blake, R and Mouton, J (1964) *The Managerial Grid.* Houston, TX: Gulf.

Bleakley, A (2006) You are who I say you are: the rhetorical construction of identity in the operating theatre. *Journal of Workplace Learning*, 17 (7): 414–425.

Bloom, BS (ed.) (1956) *Taxonomy of Educational Objectives.* New York: David McKay Company Inc.

BMA (2008) *Are You Starting a New Post?* www.bma.org.uk/employmentandcontracts/employmentcontracts/junior_doctors/juniordoctorstartinganewpost.jsp.

BMA (2009a) *The Individual Opt Out.* www.bma.org.uk/employmentandcontracts/working_arrangements/hours/ewtd/ewtdoptout.jsp

BMA (2009b) *Child Protection: A Toolkit for Doctors.* www.bma.org.uk/ethics/consent_and_capacity/childprotectiontoolkit.jsp.

BMJ Group blogs (2009) Shelia McLean on advance directives and the case of Kerrie Wooltorton. http://blogs.bmj.com/bmj/2009/10/01/sheila-mclean-on-advance-directives-and-the-case-of-kerrie-wooltorton/.

Bolitho v *City and Hackney Health Authority* (1997) www.publications.parliament.uk/pa/ld199798/ldjudgmt/jd971113/boli01.htm.

Boms, S (2009) www.alistapart.com/articles/burnout (accessed August 2010).

Bonner, S, Tremlett, M and Bell, MDD (2009) Are advance directives legally binding or simply the starting point for discussion of patients' best interests? *BMJ*, 339: 1230–1234.

Borges, NJ and Savickas, ML (2002) Personality and medical specialty choice: a literature review and integration. *Journal of Career Assessment*, 10: 362–380.

Borges, NJ, Savickas, ML and Jones, BJ (2004) Holland's theory applied to medical specialty choice. *Journal of Career Assessment*, 12: 188–206.

Brennan, N, Corrigan, O, Allard, J, Archer, J, Barnes, R, Bleakley, A, Collett, T and De Bere, SR (2010) The transition from medical student to junior doctor: today's experiences of Tomorrow's Doctors. *Medical Education*, 44: 449–458.

Brennan, TA, Leape, LL, Laird, NM, Herbert, L, Localio, AR, Lawthers, AG et al. (1991) Incidence of adverse events and negligence in hospitalised patients. *NEJM*, 324: 370–376.

Bristol Royal Infirmary Inquiry (2001) *Learning from Bristol: The Report of the Public Inquiry into Children's Heart Surgery at the Bristol Royal Infirmary 1984–1995*. London: Stationery Office. www.bristol-inquiry.org.uk/ (accessed November 2010).

British Medical Association (2008) *Second Report into Cohort Who Graduated in 2006*. www.bma.org.uk/healthcare_policy/cohort_studies/.

British Medical Association (2009) *Third Report into Cohort Who Graduated in 2006*. www.bma.org.uk/healthcare_policy/cohort_studies/.

Brown, G and Manogue, M (2001) AMEE Medical Education Guide 22: Refreshing Lecturing: a guide for lecturers. *Medical Teacher*, 23 (3): 231–244.

Buckman, R (1996) Talking to patients about cancer. *BMJ*, 313: 699–700.

BusinessBalls www.businessballs.com/timemanagement.htm (accessed 3 January 2011).

CAIPE (1997) *Interprofessional Education – A Definition*. CAIPE Bulletin. London: Centre for Advancement of Interprofessional Education.

CANMEDS Physician Competency Framework (2010) http://rcpsc.medical.org/canmeds/index.php (accessed September 2010).

Carbello, M (2007) *The Challenge of Migration and Health*. www.migrationanddevelopment.net/perspectives-positions/the-challenge-of-migration-and-health (accessed 18 February 2011).

Changing Minds http://changingminds.org/techniques/questioning/socratic_questions.htm (accessed 12 September 2010).

Cherniss, C and Goleman, D (eds) (2001) *The Emotionally Intelligent Workplace*. San Francisco: Jossey-Bass.

Chiu, LF (2003) *The Application and Management of the Community Health Educator Model: Handbook for Practitioners*. Nuffield Institute for Health, University of Leeds.

Chiu, LF (2006) Critical Reflection: More than Nuts and Bolts. *Action Research*, 4(2): 183–203.

Chiu, LF (in press) *Patient and Community Empowerment: Guidance for Migrant-Friendly and Culturally Competent Healthcare Organisation*. A draft prepared on behalf of the Working Group on Patients and Community Empowerment, The WHO-HPH International Task Force on Migrant-Friendly and Culturally Competent Hospitals May, 2006.

Coiera, E and Tombs, V (1998) Communication behaviours in a hospital setting: an observational study. *BMJ,* 316: 673–676.

Collegiate Project Services (2006) *Leadership Styles for Dealing with People – Part 1.* www.collegiateproject.com/leadershiparticles.asp (accessed October 2010).

Collins, J (2010) *Foundation for Excellence: An Evaluation of the Foundation Programme.* London: Medical Education England. www.mee.nhs.uk/pdf/401339_MEE_ FoundationExcellence_acc.pdf (Last accessed November 2010).

Colthart, I, Bagnall, G, Evans, A, Allbutt, H, Haig, A, Illing, J and McKinstry, B (2007). BEME Guide 10: A systematic review of the literature on the effectiveness of self-assessment in clinical education. *BEME Collaboration.* www2.warwick.ac.uk/ fac/med/beme/published/mckinstry/bemefinalreportsa240108.pdf (accessed 12 September 2010).

Cooper, N, Forrest, K and Cramp, P (2006) *Essential Guide to Generic Skills.* London: Blackwell Publishing.

Coulter, A (1999) Paternalism or partnership? *BMJ,* 319: 719–720.

Coulter, A (2009) *Implementing Shared Decision-Making in the UK: A Report for the Health Foundation.* London: Health Foundation.

Data Protection Act, 1998 www.legislation.gov.uk/ukpga/1998/29/contents.

Dawson, JF, Yan, X and West, MA (2007) *Positive and Negative Effects of Team Working in Healthcare: Real and Pseudo-teams and Their Impact on Safety.* Birmingham: Aston University.

Dean, B, Schachter, M, Vincent, C and Barber, N (2002) Prescribing errors in hospital inpatients: their incidence and clinical significance. *Qual Saf Health Care,* 11: 340–344.

Delbanco, T, Berwick, DM, Boufford, JI, Edgman-Levitan, S, Ollenschläger, G, Plamping, D and Rockefeller, RG (2001) Healthcare in a land called People Power: nothing about me without me. *Health Expect,* 4 (3): 144–150.

Department of Health (1989) *Working for Patients* (White Paper). London: HMSO.

Department of Health, The Caldicott Committee (1997) *Report on the Review of Patient-Identifiable Information* (The Caldicott Report). www.dh.gov.uk/en/ Publicationsandstatistics/Publications/PublicationsPolicyAndGuidance/DH_ 4068403.

Department of Health (1998) *A First Class Service – Quality in the New NHS.* London: HMSO.

Department of Health (2000) *An Organisation with a Memory: Report of an Expert Group on Learning from Adverse Events in the NHS.* London: Department of Health. www.dh.gov.uk

Department of Health (2004) *Choosing Health: Making Healthy Choices Easier.* Command Paper 6374. http://webarchive.nationalarchives.gov.uk/+/www.dh.gov.

uk/en/Publicationsandstatistics/Publications/PublicationsPolicyAndGuidance/
DH_4094550.

Department of Health (2009) *Legal Issues Relevant to Non-heartbeating Organ Donation*.
www.dh.gov.uk/en/Publicationsandstatistics/Publications/PublicationsPolicyAnd
Guidance/DH_108825

Department of Health (2010a) *Equity and Excellence: Liberating the NHS*. White Paper
Cm 7881. www.dh.gov.uk/en/Publicationsandstatistics/Publications/PublicationsP
olicyAndGuidance/DH_117353.

Department of Health (2010b) *Liberating the NHS: Report of the Arms-Length Bodies
Review*. www.dh.gov.uk/prod_consum_dh/groups/dh_digitalassets/@dh/@en/@
ps/documents/digitalasset/dh_118053.pdf.

Department of Health and Social Security (1980) *Inequalities in Health: Report of a
Research Working Group* (Black Report). London: DHSS. www.sochealth.co.uk/
history/black.htm.

Dewey, J (1897) My pedagogic creed. *School Journal*, 54 (January): 77–80. http://
dewey.pragmatism.org/creed.htm (accessed 13 September 2010).

Directgov *Working Time Limits: The 48 Hour Week* www.direct.gov.uk/en/
Employment/Employees/WorkingHoursAndTimeOff/DG_10029426

Donabedian, A. (1988) Quality assessment and assurance unity of purpose, diversity
of means. *Inquiry*, 25: 173–192.

Drucker, PF (1993) *The Effective Executive*. New York: HarperBusiness.

Eng, E, Parker, EA and Harlan, C (1997) Lay health advisors: A critical link to community capacity building (special issue). *Health Education and Behavior*, 24 (4): 407–526.

Epstein, RM (1999) Mindful practice. *JAMA*, 282 (9): 833–839.

Eraut, M (1994) *Developing Professional Knowledge and Competence*. London: Falmer
Press.

Eraut, M (2000) Non-formal learning, implicit learning and tacit knowledge in
professional work in Coffield, F. (ed.), *The Necessity of Informal Learning*. Bristol: The
Policy Press.

Fallowfield, L and Jenkins, V (2004) Communicating sad, bad, and difficult news in
medicine. *Lancet*, 363: 312–319.

Fitzpatrick, R (1996) Telling patients nothing is wrong. *BMJ*, 313: 311–312.

Foundation Programme. www.foundationprogramme.nhs.uk/pages/home
(accessed 11 August 2010).

Fox, M (2010) *US Apologises for Syphilis Experiment in Guatemala*. Reuters. http://
uk.reuters.com/article/idUKTRE6903RZ20101001.

Gawande, A (2010) *The Checklist Manifesto – How to Get Things Right*. London: Profile
Books.

General Medical Council (1999) *Doctor as Teacher*. Archived policy document. www.gmc-uk.org/education/postgraduate/doctor_as_teacher.asp (accessed 13 September 2010).

General Medical Council (2006) *Good Medical Practice*. London: General Medical Council. www.gmc-uk.org (accessed 6 September 2009).

General Medical Council (2006a) *Management for Doctors*. London: General Medical Council.

General Medical Council (2008) *Personal Beliefs and Medical Practice: Guidance for Doctors*. www.gmc-uk.org/guidance/ethical_guidance/personal_beliefs.asp.

General Medical Council (2009a) *Tomorrow's Doctors*. London: General Medical Council. www.gmc-uk.org/education/undergraduate/undergraduate_policy/tomorrows_doctors/tomorrows_doctors_2009.asp (accessed 6 September 2009).

General Medical Council (2009b) *Confidentiality*. www.gmc-uk.org/Confidentiality_core_2009.pdf_27494212.pdf (accessed August 2010).

General Medical Council (2009c) *Good Medical Practice*. www.gmc-uk.org/guidance/good_medical_practice/duties_of_a_doctor.asp.

General Medical Council (2009d) *The New Doctor*. www.gmc-uk.org/New_Doctor09_FINAL.pdf_27493417.pdf.

General Medical Council (2010a) *Medical Students and Fitness to Practice*. www.gmc-uk.org/education/undergraduate/professional_behaviour.asp.

General Medical Council (2010b) *Treatment and Care Towards the End of Life*. London: GMC.

General Medical Council (2010c) *Workplace Based Assessment: A Guide for Implementation*. www.gmc-uk.org/Workplace_Based_Assessment.pdf_31300577.pdf (accessed 11 August 2010).

General Medical Council (2010d) GMC *Education Strategy 2011–2013: Shaping the Future of Medical Education and Training*. www.gmc-uk.org/Education_Strategy_2011_2013.pdf_36672939.pdf.

General Medical Council (2010e) *Generic Standards for Speciality Including GP Training*. www.gmc-uk.org/Generic_standards_for_specialty_including_GP_training_Oct_2010.pdf_35788108.pdf_39279982.pdf.

General Medical Council (2010f) *Determination on Serious Professional Misconduct (SPM) and Sanction*. Online: www.gmc-uk.org/Wakefield_SPM_and_SANCTION.pdf_32595267.pdf.

General Medical Council (2011). *Good Medical Practice*. www.gmc-uk.org/guidance/good_medical_practice.asp.

Gill, P, Kai, J, Bhopl, R and Wild, S (2007) Health Care Needs Assessment: The epidemiologically based needs assessment review: Black and Minority Groups. *Black and Minority Groups*. Birmingham: University of Birmingham.

Goldacre, MJ, Turner, G and Lambert, TW (2004) Variation by medical school in career choices of UK graduates of 1999 and 2000. *Medical Education*, 38: 249–258.

Goldacre, MJ, Laxton L and Lambert, TW (2010) Medical graduates' early career choices of specialty and their eventual specialty destinations: UK prospective cohort studies. *British Medical Journal*, doi:10.1136/bmj.c3199.

Goleman, D (1998) *Working with Emotional Intelligence*. London: Bloomsbury.

Goleman, D (2000) Leadership that gets results. *Harvard Business Review*, 7 (2): 78–90.

Good, BJ, Herrera, H, Good, DelVecchio, M-J and Cooper, J (1985) Reflexivity, countertransference and clinical ethnography: a case from a psychiatric cultural consultation clinic, in Hahn, RA and Gaines, AD (eds) *Physicians of Western Medicine*. Dordrecht: Reidel, 193–221.

Greenleaf, RK (1977) *Servant Leadership: A Journey into the Nature of Legitimate Power and Greatness*. New Jersey: Paulist Press.

Gregg, MF and Magilvy, JK (2001) Professional identity of Japanese nurses: bonding into nursing. *Nursing and Health Sciences*, 3 (1), 47–55.

Gruen, R and Howarth, A (2005) *Financial Management in Health Services*, Maidenhead, Berks: Open University Press.

Gunderman, R (2009) *Leadership in Healthcare*. London: Springer-Verlag.

Guyatt, G, Cairns, J, Churchill, D and others [Evidence-Based Medicine Working Group] Evidence-based medicine. A new approach to teaching the practice of medicine. *JAMA*, 268: 2420–2425.

Hammick, M, Freeth, D, Copperman, J and Goodsman, D (2009) *Being Interprofessional*. Cambridge: Polity.

Hassan, R, Kanoum, K and Cooper, N (2009) Team Communication on the Acute Medical Unit. Poster. Society for Acute Medicine 3rd International Conference, Birmingham, October.

Health Protection Agency, HPA Standards. www.hpa.org.uk/web/HPAweb&HPAwebStandard/HPAweb_C/1238230848780.

Heinreich, HW, Peterson, D and Roos, N (1980) *Industrial Accident Prevention* (5th edition). New York: McGraw-Hill.

Helman, CG (1994) *Culture, Health and Illness*. Oxford: Butterworth-Heinemann.

Henderson, M (2009) Cardiologist will fight libel case 'to defend free speech', *The Times*, 26 November. http://business.timesonline.co.uk/tol/business/law/article6932252.ece.

Hirsh, W, Jackson, C and Kidd, J (2001) *Straight Talking: Effective Career Discussions at Work*. Cambridge: National Institute for Careers Education and Counselling.

HM Treasury (2004) *Securing Good Health for the Whole Population, Final Report* (Wanless Report). http://webarchive.nationalarchives.gov.uk/+/www.dh.gov.

uk/en/Publichealth/Healthinequalities/Healthinequalitiesguidancepublications/
DH_066213.

Horsburgh, M, Perkins, R, Coyle, B and Degeling, P (2006) The professional subcultures of students entering medicine, nursing and pharmacy programmes. *Journal of Interprofessional Care*, 20 (4): 425–431.

Hutson, P and Rowan, M (1998) Qualitative studies: their role in medical research. *Canadian Family Physician*, 44: 2453–2458.

Illing, J, Peile, E, Morrison, J and Morrow, G (2008) *How Prepared Are Medical Graduates to Begin Practice? A Comparison of Three Diverse UK Medical Schools*. London: GMC.

Imison, C and Giordano, RW (2009) Doctors as leaders. *British Medical Journal*, 338: 979–980.

Infed Encyclopaedia of informal learning. www.infed.org/ (accessed 11 August 2010).Information Commissioner's Office (ICO). Guide to data protection – definitions, principles and practical examples. www.ico.gov.uk/for_organisations/data_protection/the_guide.aspx (accessed 20 April 2011)

Institute for Healthcare Improvement (2005) *Going Lean in Health Care.* IHI Innovation Series white paper. Cambridge, MA: Institute for Healthcare Improvement. www.IHI.org.

Jackson, C, Hirsh, W and Kidd, J (2003) *Informing Choices. The Need for Careers Advice in Medical Training*. Cambridge: National Institute for Careers Education and Counselling.

Jones, L (undated) personal communication about models of reflection ('I, we, they' cycle).

Kelley, RE (1992) *The Power of Followership: How to Create Leaders People Want to Follow and Followers Who Lead Themselves.* New York: Currency Doubleday.

Kernick, D (2010) Leading in complex environments, in Swanwick, T and McKimm, J (eds) *The ABC of Clinical Leadership*. Oxford: Wiley Blackwell.

Knowles, M (1983) *The Adult Learner: A Neglected Species*. Houston: Gulf.

Kolb, D (1984) *Experiential Learning*. Englewood Cliffs: Prentice Hall.

Kraft, U (2006) The burnout cycle. *Scientific American Mind*, 17 (3).

Lang, F, Floyd, MR and Beine, KL (2000) Clues to patients' explanations and concerns about their illnesses. *Arch Fam Med*, 9 (3): 222–227.

Langewitz, W, Denz, M, Keller, A, Kiss, A, Rutimann, S and Wossmer, B (2002) Spontaneous talking time at start of consultation in outpatient clinic: cohort study. *BMJ*, 325, 682 doi: 10.1136/bmj.325.7366.682.

Langley, G, Nolan, K, Nolan, T, Norman, C and Provost, L (1996) *The Improvement Guide: A Practical Approach to Enhancing Organisational Performance*. San Francisco: Jossey Bass.

Lave, J and Wenger, E (1991) *Situated Learning: Legitimate Peripheral Participation*. Cambridge: Cambridge University Press.

Leape, LL (1994) The preventability of medical injury, in Bogner, MS (ed.) *Human Error in Medicine*. Hillsdale, NJ: Lawrence Erlbaum Associates.

Leeds Teaching Hospitals NHS Trust (LTHT) (2002) *Report of the Independent Inquiry into the Colin Norris Incidents at Leeds Teaching Hospitals NHS Trust (LTHT) in 2002*. www.leeds.nhs.uk/Default.aspx.LocID-0ernew02s.RefLocID-0er00q001. Lang-EN.htm

Lewin, SA, Dick, J, Pond, P, Zwarenstein, M, et al. (2006) Lay health workers in primary and community health care. *The Cochrane Database of Systematic Reviews* (31 March), 1. www.cochrane.org/reviews/en/ab004015.

Lingard, L, Garwood, K, Schryer, CF and Spafford, M (2003) A certain art of uncertainty: case presentation and the development of professional identity. *Social Science and Medicine*, 56 (3): 603–616.

Lister, S (1996) Approaches to Audit. *Audit in General Practice*, 4 (3): 6–7.

London Deanery. *Faculty Development: E-learning Modules for Clinical Teachers*. www.faculty.londondeanery.ac.uk/e-learning/ (accessed 11 August 2010).

Maguire, P (2000) *Communication Skills for Doctors*. London: Arnold.

Marmot, M (2010) *Fair Society, Healthy Lives: Strategic Review of Health Inequalities in England – Post 2010*. www.marmotreview.org/.

Marmot, M and Wilkinson, R (2006) *The Social Determinants of Health*, 2nd edition. Oxford: Oxford University Press.

Maslach, C, Jackson, SE and Leiter, MP (1996) *MBI: The Maslach Burnout Inventory: Manual*. Palo Alto: Consulting Psychologists Press.

Maxwell, RJ (1984) Quality assessment in health. *British Medical Journal*, 288: 1470–1472.

Mayo, WJ (1928) *The aims and ideals of the American Medical Association*, address given at the 66th Annual Meeting of the National Education Association, Minneapolis, 1–6 July 1928. www.allthingswilliam.com/medicine.html (9 September 2010).

Mazzocato, P, Savage, C, Brommels, M, Aronsson, H and Thor, J (2010) Lean thinking in healthcare: a realist review of the literature. *Quality and Safety in Health Care*, 19 (5): 376–382.

McAllister, B (1997) *Crew Resource Management: Awareness, Cockpit Efficiency and Safety*. Shrewsbury: Airlife Publishing Ltd.

McKimm, J and Swanwick, T (2010) Assessing learning needs, in McKimm, J and Swanwick, T (eds) *Clinical Teaching Made Easy*. London: Quay Books.

McPherson, W (1999) *The Stephen Lawrence Inquiry: Report on an Inquiry by Sir William*

McPherson on CLUNY, presented to the Parliament by Secretary of State for the Home Department by command of Her Majesty.

McQuillan, P, Pilkington S, Allan A, Taylor B, Short A, Morgan G, et al. (1998) Confidential inquiry into quality of care before admission to intensive care. *BMJ*, 316: 1853–1858.

Medical Protection Society. www.medicalprotection.org/uk/education (accessed September 2010).

Mercer, SW and Reynolds, WJ (2002) Empathy and quality of care. *British Journal of General Practice (Quality Supplement)*, 52: S9–S13.

Mercer, SW, McConnachie, A, Maxwell, M, Heaney, DH and Watt, GCM (2005) Relevance and performance of the Consultation and Relational Empathy (CARE) Measure in general practice. *Family Practice*, 22 (3): 328–334.

Mills, AJ and Ransom, K (2001) The design of health systems, in Merson, MH, Black, RE and Mills, AJ (eds) *International Public Health: Diseases, Programs, Systems and Policies*, Gaithersburg, MD: Aspen.

Moulton, L (2007) *The Naked Consultation*. Oxford: Radcliffe Medical Press.

National Association of Clinical Tutors (2008) *Managing Trainees in Difficulty: Practical Advice for Educational and Clinical Supervisors*. www.nact.org.uk/pdf_documents/nactdocs/Trainees%20in%20Difficulty%20Jan%2008.pdf (accessed August 2010).

National Clinical Assessment Service (NCAS) (2010) www.ncas.npsa.nhs.uk/ (accessed August 2010).

National Patient Safety Agency (2004) *Seven Steps to Patient Safety*. www.nrls.npsa.nhs.uk/resources/collections/seven-steps-to-patient-safety/?entryid45=59787 (accessed September 2010).

Neighbour, R (2005) *The Inner Consultation*, 2nd edition. Oxford: Radcliffe Medical Press.

Nelson, G, Batalden, P, Plume, S and Mohr, J (1996) Improving Health Care Part 2 – A Clinical Improvement Worksheet and Users' Manual. *The Joint Commission Journal on Quality Improvement*, 22 (8): 531–548.

NHS (2010) *Gold Guide to Specialty Training*. www.mmc.nhs.uk.

NHS Careers (2010) *Welcome to the Medical Team*. www.nhsemployers.org/SiteCollectionDocuments/Junior%20doctor%202009%20final.pdf.

NHS Institute for Innovation and Improvement (2007) *The Improvement Leaders' Guides*. www.institute.nhs.uk/improvementleadersguide.

NHS Institute for Innovation and Improvement (2010) The SBAR model. www.institute.nhs.uk/safer_care/safer_care/Situation_Background_Assessment_Recommendation.html (accessed December 2010).

NHS Institute of Innovation and Improvement and Academy of Royal Colleges (2008) *Medical Leadership Competency Framework*. www.institute.nhs.uk/assessment_tool/general/medical_leadership_competency_framework_-_homepage.html (accessed 5 September 2009).

NHS Institute of Innovation and Improvement and Academy of Royal Colleges (2010) *Medical Leadership Competency Framework*. www.institute.nhs.uk/assessment_tool/general/medical_leadership_competency_framework_-_homepage.html (accessed 19 August 2010).

NICE (National Institute for Clinical Excellence) (2002) *Guidance on the Use of Ultrasound Locating Devices for Placing Central Venous Catheters*. Technology appraisal Guidance – No. 49. September.

Patient Voices Programme. www.patientvoices.org.uk/. Last accessed 11 August 2010.

Pedler, M (2001) *A Manager's Guide to Self-development*. Maidenhead: McGraw-Hill International (UK) Ltd.

Pendleton, D, Schofield, T, Tate, P and Havelock, P (2003) *The New Consultation: Developing Doctor-Patient Communication*. Oxford: Oxford University Press.

Perkins, HS (2007) Controlling death: the false promise of advance directives. *Ann Intern Med*, 147: 51–57.

Picker Institute Europe and Care Quality Commission. NHS Surveys. www.nhssurveys.org/publications (accessed September 2010).

Plsek, PE and Greenhalgh, T (2001) Complexity science: the challenge of complexity in health care. *British Medical Journal*, 323: 625–628.

Popper, K (2002/1935) *The Logic of Scientific Discovery*, 2nd edition. Taylor & Francis E-library.

Pothier, D, Monteiro, P, Mooktiar, M and Shaw, A (2005) Pilot study to show the loss of important data in nursing handover. *British Journal of Nursing*, 14 (20): 1090–1093.

Preston-Shoot, M and McKimm, J (2010) Prepared for practice? Law teaching and assessment in UK medical schools. *Journal of Medical Ethics*, 36, 694–699.

Preston-Shoot, M, McKimm, J, Kong, WM and Smith, S. (in press) Readiness for legally literate medical practice? Student perceptions of their undergraduate medico-legal education. *Journal of Medical Ethics*.

Reason, J (2000) Human error: models and management. *BMJ*, 320: 768–767.

Reason, J (2006) Conference presentation, Association for the Study of Medical Education (ASME), Aberdeen, July.

Ridd, M, Shaw, A, Lewis, G and Salisbury, C (2009) The patient–doctor relationship: a systematic review of the qualitative literature on patients' perspectives. *BJGP*, 59: 268–275.

Roemer, MI (1991) *National Health Systems of the World, Volume 1: The Countries.* Oxford: Oxford University Press.

Roter, D (2000) The enduring and evolving nature of the patient-physician relationship. *Patient Education and Counseling*, 39: 5–15.

Royal College of Physicians (1997) *Improving Communication between Doctors and Patients: A Report of a Working Party.* London: RCP.

Royal College of Physicians (2005) *Doctors in Society: Medical Professionalism in a Changing World: Report of a Working Party of the Royal College of Physicians.* London: RCP.

Royal College Physicians (2006) *Explaining the Risks and Benefits of Treatment Options: Suggestions for Hospital Doctors. PIU information sheet 1.* Online: www.rcplondon.ac.uk.

Sackett, SL, Rosenberg, WC, Gray, JAM, et al. (1996) Evidence based medicine: what it is and what it isn't. *BMJ*, 312: 71–72.

Sari, AB, Sheldon, TA, Cracknell, A, Turnbull, A, Dobson, Y, Grant, C, Gray, W and Richardson, A (2007) Extent, nature and consequences of adverse events: results of a retrospective case note review in a large NHS hospital. *Qual Saf Health Care*, 16: 434–439.

Savulescu, J (2006) Conscientious objection in medicine. *BMJ*, 332: 294–297.

Schön, D (1983) *The Reflective Practitioner: Towards a New Design for Teaching and Learning in the Professions.* San Francisco: Jossey Bass.

SDO Briefing Paper (2006) *Achieving High Performance in Health Care Systems: The Impact and Influence of Organizational Arrangements.* London: NHS Service Delivery and Organization Research Programme.

Sfard, A. (1988) On two metaphors for learning and the danger of choosing just one. *Educational Researcher*, 27: 4–13.

Silverman, J, Kurtz, S and Draper, J (2005) *Skills for Communicating with Patients*, 2nd edition. Oxford: Radcliffe Medical Press.

Spiro, H (1992) *Empathy and the Practice of Medicine: Beyond Pills and the Scalpel.* London: Yale University Press.

Stavropoulou, C (2010) Non-adherence to medication and doctor–patient relationship: evidence from a European survey. *Pat Education and Counseling*, doi:10.1016/j.pec.2010.04.039.

Stewart, J (2007) 'Don't hesitate to call' – the underlying assumptions. *The Clinical Teacher*, 4: 6–9.

Stewart, M, Belle Brown, J, Wayne Weston, W, McWhinney, IR, McWilliam, C and Freeman, T (2003) *Patient-Centred Medicine: Transforming the Clinical Method*, 2nd edition. Oxford: Radcliffe Medical Press.

Smiles, S (1866) *Self Help*. London: John Murray.

Straus, SE, Glasziou, P, Richardson, WS and Haynes, RB (2010) *Evidence-Based*

Medicine: How to Practice and Teach It, 4th edition. Oxford: Churchill Livingstone, Elsevier Publishing.

Suchman, AL, Markakis, K, Beckman, HB and Frankel R (1997) A model of empathic communication in the medical interview. *JAMA*, 277 (8): 678–682.

Swanwick, T and Morris, C (2010) Shifting conceptions of learning in the workplace. *Medical Education*, 44 (6): 538–539.

Thistlethwaite, JE and Spencer, J (2009) *Professionalism in Medicine.* Abingdon: Radcliffe Medical Press.

Thistlethwaite, JE and Moran, M (2010). Learning outcomes for interprofessional education (IPE): literature review and synthesis. *Journal of Interprofessional Care*, 24: 503–513.

The Times (2004) Right to life: should a doctor or a lawyer guard death's door? Editorial, 31 July.

Tochel, C, Haig, A, Hesketh, A, Cadzow, A, Beggs, K, Colthart, I and Peacock, H (2009) The effectiveness of portfolios for post-graduate assessment and education: BEME Guide No 12. *Medical Teacher*, 31: 320–339.

Tooke, J (2008) *Aspiring to Excellence*: *Final Report of the Independent Inquiry into Modernising Medical Careers*. www.mmcinquiry.org.uk.

Travers, KD (1997) Reducing inequities through participatory research and community empowerment. *Health Education and Behaviour*, 24: 344–356.

Travis, JS and Ryan, RS (2004) *Wellness Workbook*, 3rd edition. Berkeley: Ten Speed Press.

Trivedi, D, Sherminder, S and Hooke, R (2008) *British Journal of Hospital Medicine*, 69 (10 MMC Supp): M150 – M151 (Oct).

UK Foundation Programme Office (2010) *The Foundation Programme Curriculum*. Cardiff: UK Foundation Programme Office. www.foundationprogramme.nhs.uk/pages/home (accessed 6 September 2009).

UK Foundation Programme Office (2008) *Rough Guide to the Academic Foundation Programme*. Cardiff: UK Foundation Programme Office. www.foundationprogramme.nhs.uk/pages/home (accessed 6 September 2009).

UK Foundation Programme Office (2009) *Compendium of Academic Competences*. Cardiff: UK Foundation Programme Office. www.foundationprogramme.nhs.uk/pages/home/key-documents (accessed 19 August 2010).

UK Foundation Programme Office (2009a) *Compendium of Academic Competencies*. www.foundationprogramme.nhs.uk/download.asp?file=Compendium_of_Academic_Competences.pdf.

UK Foundation Programme Office (2010) *The Foundation Programme Reference Guide*. Cardiff: UK Foundation Programme Office. www.foundationprogramme.nhs.uk/pages/home/key-documents (accessed 19 August 2010).

Vandekieft, GK (2001) Breaking bad news. *American Family Physician*, 64: 1975–1978. www.aafp.org/afp/20011215/1975.pdf (accessed November 2010).

Veloski, J, Boex, J, Grasberger, J, Evans, A and Wolfson, B (2006) Systematic review of the literature on assessment, feedback and physicians' clinical performance? BEME Guide No. 7. *Medical Teacher*, 28 (2): 117–128.

Vincent, C, Neale, G and Woloshynowych, M (2001) Adverse event in British hospitals: preliminary retrospective record review. *BMJ*, 322: 517–519.

Wallerstein, N (1992). Powerlessness, empowerment, and health: implications for health promotion programs. *American Journal of Health Promotion*, 6 (3): 197–205.

Washer, P (ed) (2009) *Clinical Communication Skills*. Oxford: Oxford University Press.

Weinman, J, Yusuf, G, Berks, R, Rayner, S and Petrie, KJ (2009) How accurate is patients' anatomical knowledge: a cross-sectional, questionnaire study of six patient groups and a general public sample. *BMC Family Practice*, 10:43doi:10.1186/1471-2296-10-43.

Wilson, TD (2009) Knowing me, myself and I: what psychology can contribute to self-knowledge. *Perspectives on Psychological Science*, Association for Psychological Science (2009, September 8)

Wilson, RM, Runciman, WB, Gibberd, RW, Harrison, BT, Newby, L and Hamilton, JD (1995) The quality in Australian healthcare study. *Medical Journal of Australia*, 163: 458–471.

Wong, MC, Yee, KC and Turner, P (2008) *Clinical Handover Literature Review, eHealth Services Research Group, University of Tasmania Australia*. www.safetyandquality.gov.au/internet/ safety/publishing.nsf/Content/PriorityProgram-05.

World Alliance for Patient Safety (2008) *WHO Surgical Safety Checklist and Implementation Manual.* www.who.int/patientsafety/safesurgery/ss_checklist/en/index.html (accessed September 2010).

World Health Organisation [WHO] (1986) *The Ottawa Charter for Health Promotion.* Charter adopted on November 17–21, 1986 Ottawa, Ontario, Canada.

World Health Organisation [WHO] (2005) *The Bangkok Charter for Health Promotion in a Globalised World.* Charter produced at the 6th Global Conference on Health Promotion, 11 August 2005, Bangkok, Thailand.

World Health Organisation [WHO] (2009) *Framework for Action on Interprofessional Education and Collaborative Practice.* Geneva: WHO.

Yukl, G (2002) *Leadership in Organisations* (5th edition). New Jersey: Prentice Hall.

Index